AIDS/HIV

ISSN 1532-2718

AIDS/HIV

Barbara Wexler

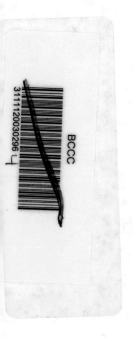

INFORMATION PLUS® REFERENCE SERIES
Formerly published by Information Plus, Wylie, Texas

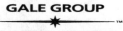
GALE GROUP
THOMSON LEARNING

Detroit • New York • San Diego • San Francisco
Boston • New Haven, Conn. • Waterville, Maine
London • Munich

AIDS/HIV

Barbara Wexler, *Author*

The Gale Group Staff:
Coordinating Editors: Ellice Engdahl, *Series Editor;* Charles B. Montney, *Series Graphics Editor*
Managing Editor: Debra M. Kirby
Contributing Editors: Elizabeth Manar, Kathleen Meek
Contributing Associate Editors: Paula Cutcher-Jackson, Prindle LaBarge, Heather Price, Michael T. Reade
Imaging and Multimedia Content: Barbara J. Yarrow, Manager, *Imaging and Multimedia Content;* Dean Dauphinais, *Imaging and Multimedia Content Editor;* Kelly A. Quin, *Imaging and Multimedia Content Editor;* Robyn Young, *Imaging and Multimedia Content Editor;* Leitha Etheridge-Sims, *Image Cataloger;* Mary K. Grimes, *Image Cataloger;* David G. Oblender, *Image Cataloger*; Lezlie Light, *Imaging Coordinator*; Randy Bassett, *Imaging Supervisor*; Robert Duncan, *Imaging Specialist*; Dan Newell, *Imaging Specialist*; Luke Rademacher, *Imaging Specialist*; Christine O'Bryan, *Graphic Specialist*
Indexing: Susan Kelsch, *Indexing Supervisor*
Permissions: Lori Hines, *Permissions Assistant*; Maria Franklin, *Permissions Manager*
Product Design: Michelle DiMercurio, *Senior Art Director and Product Design Manager*; Michael Logusz, *Graphic Artist*
Production: Evi Seoud, *Assistant Manager, Composition Purchasing and Electronic Prepress*; Keith Helmling, *Buyer*; Dorothy Maki, *Manufacturing Manager*
Cover photo © Digital Stock.

TABLE OF CONTENTS

In the year 2000 HIV was the fifth leading cause of death among those aged 25–44. This chapter investigates the nature of HIV/AIDS, including an in-depth look at the HIV virus, its origins, how it attacks the immune system, and the search for answers. Diseases associated with HIV infection, such as tuberculosis and cancer, are also covered.

The first section of Chapter 2 defines AIDS and examines the Centers for Disease Control and Prevention's classification revision and expanded case surveillance. A second section details the diagnosis and symptoms of AIDS, transmission, and the safety of blood transfusions and transplant procedures. Information about testing for HIV and tracking the progress of HIV to full-blown AIDS is also included.

AIDS is infecting an increasingly diverse population. Once thought to affect only homosexual males and intravenous drug users, AIDS is now occurring in women and those in heterosexual contact. Chapter 3 explores AIDS case numbers, including regional differences and the growing incidence of AIDS in women. This chapter also discusses HIV transmittal and life expectancy of a person infected with HIV/AIDS.

It had previously been thought that certain populations were at greater risk for contracting HIV/AIDS. This chapter focuses on the rates of HIV/AIDS in various populations, including heterosexuals, intravenous drug users, and women. Special coverage is given to hemophiliacs and prisoners.

HIV/AIDS in children is different than HIV/AIDS in adults. This chapter explains why by presenting a case definition, a discussion of the number of children infected, and how children acquire HIV/AIDS. The remainder of the chapter explores adolescents and AIDS, detailing such issues as transmission by sexually active teens.

Care for HIV/AIDS patients is expensive: a person with AIDS could spend approximately $77,000 a year on medications. This chapter tracks AIDS health-care financing, covering such issues as state programs to provide drugs; costs to the insurance industry; and challenges to the delivery systems of hospitals, physicians' offices, and direct-care staff. A special section pertaining to health-care workers and HIV/AIDS is also included.

In 2000 it was estimated that the federal government spent approximately $11 billion on HIV-related expenses. The costs of treatment and research are investigated in this chapter. Special emphasis is given to FDA-approved drugs, the recent discovery of an HIV-resistant gene, new research, and the search for a vaccine.

Now, more than ever, Americans are likely to know of someone with HIV/AIDS. Chapter 8 focuses on celebrities, such as Earvin "Magic" Johnson, and older people with AIDS. Problems such as depression, suicide, and housing are also considered.

Few issues about HIV/AIDS inspire as much controversy as HIV testing. This chapter discusses HIV-testing in terms of mandatory versus voluntary testing, and partner notification. Other areas covered are educating youth; condom use; and improving prevention programs. Intravenous drug users and syringe exchange programs are given special attention.

HIV/AIDS has become a global problem. Chapter 10 investigates the scope of the global HIV/AIDS pandemic, covering such areas as global trends and projections; the effect of AIDS on birth and death rates; patterns of infection; and the difference between HIV-1 and HIV-2. The status of HIV/AIDS in Africa, Europe, Asia, Latin America, the Caribbean, and the Middle East is also updated.

PREFACE

AIDS/HIV is one of the latest volumes in the Information Plus Reference Series. Previously published by the Information Plus company of Wylie, Texas, the Information Plus Reference Series (and its companion set, the Information Plus Compact Series) became a Gale Group product when Gale and Information Plus merged in early 2000. Those of you familiar with the series as published by Information Plus will notice a few changes from the 2000 edition. Gale has adopted a new layout and style that we hope you will find easy to use. Other improvements include greatly expanded indexes in each book, and more descriptive tables of contents.

While some changes have been made to the design, the purpose of the Information Plus Reference Series remains the same. Each volume of the series presents the latest facts on a topic of pressing concern in modern American life. These topics include today's most controversial and most studied social issues: abortion, capital punishment, care for the elderly, crime, health care, the environment, immigration, minorities, social welfare, women, youth, and many more. Although written especially for the high school and undergraduate student, this series is an excellent resource for anyone in need of factual information on current affairs.

By presenting the facts, it is Gale's intention to provide its readers with everything they need to reach an informed opinion on current issues. To that end, there is a particular emphasis in this series on the presentation of scientific studies, surveys, and statistics. These data are generally presented in the form of tables, charts, and other graphics placed within the text of each book. Every graphic is directly referred to and carefully explained in the text. The source of each graphic is presented within the graphic itself. The data used in these graphics are drawn from the most reputable and reliable sources, in particular the various branches of the U.S. government and major independent polling organizations. Every

effort has been made to secure the most recent information available. The reader should bear in mind that many major studies take years to conduct, and that additional years often pass before the data from these studies are made available to the public. Therefore, in many cases the most recent information available in 2002 dated from 1999 or 2000. Older statistics are sometimes presented as well, if they are of particular interest and no more recent information exists.

Although statistics are a major focus of the Information Plus Reference Series, they are by no means its only content. Each book also presents the widely held positions and important ideas that shape how the book's subject is discussed in the United States. These positions are explained in detail and, where possible, in the words of their proponents. Some of the other material to be found in these books includes: historical background; descriptions of major events related to the subject; relevant laws and court cases; and examples of how these issues play out in American life. Some books also feature primary documents, or have pro and con debate sections giving the words and opinions of prominent Americans on both sides of a controversial topic. All material is presented in an even-handed and unbiased manner; the reader will never be encouraged to accept one view of an issue over another.

HOW TO USE THIS BOOK

The spread of AIDS has become a global epidemic. As of 2000, 36.1 million people worldwide were living with AIDS. In that same year, HIV infection was the fifth leading cause of death among persons aged 25–44 in America. This book provides a snapshot of HIV/AIDS in the United States. Included is information on the nature of HIV/AIDS and the AIDS epidemic; symptoms and transmittal; populations at risk; children, adolescents, and HIV/AIDS; HIV/AIDS and the health-care system; cost, treatment, and research; testing, prevention, and education; HIV and

AIDS worldwide; and knowledge, behavior, and opinion of those affected by AIDS/HIV.

AIDS/HIV consists of eleven chapters and three appendices. Each of the chapters is devoted to a particular aspect of AIDS/HIV. For a summary of the information covered in each chapter, please see the synopses provided in the Table of Contents at the front of the book. Chapters generally begin with an overview of the basic facts and background information on the chapter's topic, then proceed to examine sub-topics of particular interest. For example, Chapter Two: Definition, Symptoms, and Transmittal begins with a definition of AIDS and an explanation of the 1993 classification revision and expanded surveillance case definition. It then goes on to provide information about the diagnosis and symptoms of AIDS, transmission, safety of blood and transplant procedures, and testing for HIV (including diagnostic, urine, and home tests). Readers can find their way through a chapter by looking for the section and subsection headings, which are clearly set off from the text. Or, they can refer to the book's extensive index if they already know what they are looking for.

Statistical Information

The tables and figures featured throughout *AIDS/HIV* will be of particular use to the reader in learning about this issue. These tables and figures represent an extensive collection of the most recent and important statistics on AIDS/HIV, as well as related issues—for example, graphics in the book cover fifteen leading causes of death for the total population; clinical categories of AIDS infection; adult and adolescent HIV infection and AIDS cases; confirmed AIDS cases, 1995–1999; pediatric AIDS cases; office visits, by diagnostic and screening services ordered or provided; research-based pharmaceutical and industry R&D spending; distribution of the number of patients assisted in suicide; states with confidential HIV reporting; adults and children estimated to be living with HIV/AIDS as of the end of 2000; and teens' concerns about becoming infected with HIV/AIDS. Gale believes that making this information available to the reader is the most impor-

tant way in which we fulfill the goal of this book: to help readers understand the issues and controversies surrounding AIDS/HIV in the United States and reach their own conclusions.

Each table or figure has a unique identifier appearing above it, for ease of identification and reference. Titles for the tables and figures explain their purpose. At the end of each table or figure, the original source of the data is provided.

In order to help readers understand these often complicated statistics, all tables and figures are explained in the text. References in the text direct the reader to the relevant statistics. Furthermore, the contents of all tables and figures are fully indexed. Please see the opening section of the index at the back of this volume for a description of how to find tables and figures within it.

In addition to the main body text and images, *AIDS/HIV* has three appendices. The first is the Important Names and Addresses directory. Here the reader will find contact information for a number of government and private organizations that can provide information on AIDS/HIV. The second appendix is the Resources section, which can also assist the reader in conducting his or her own research. In this section, the author and editors of *AIDS/HIV* describe some of the sources that were most useful during the compilation of this book. The final appendix is the index. It has been greatly expanded from previous editions, and should make it even easier to find specific topics in this book.

COMMENTS AND SUGGESTIONS

The editors of the Information Plus Reference Series welcome your feedback on *AIDS/HIV*. Please direct all correspondence to:

Editors
Information Plus Reference Series
27500 Drake Rd.
Farmington Hills, MI 48331-3535

ACKNOWLEDGEMENTS

The editors wish to thank the copyright holders of material included in this volume and the permissions managers of many book and magazine publishing companies for assisting us in securing reproduction rights. We are also grateful to the staffs of the Detroit Public Library, the Library of Congress, the University of Detroit Mercy Library, Wayne State University Purdy/Kresge Library Complex, and the University of Michigan Libraries for making their resources available to us.

Following is a list of the copyright holders who have granted us permission to reproduce material in Information Plus: AIDS/HIV. *Every effort has been made to trace copyright, but if omissions have been made, please let us know.*

Acknowledgements are listed in the order the tables and figures appear in the text of AIDS/HIV. For more detailed citations, please see the sources listed under each table and figure.

Table 1.1. Minino, Arialdi M. and Betty L. Smith. "Table 7. Deaths and death rates for the 10 leading causes of death in specified age groups: United States, preliminary 2000," in *Deaths: Preliminary Data for 2000, National Vital Statistics Reports*, v. 49, n. 12. National Center for Health Statistics, Hyattsville, MD.

Table 1.2. "Table C. Percent of total deaths, death rates, age-adjusted death rates for 1999, percent change in age-adjusted death rates from 1998 to 1999 and ratio of age-adjusted death rates by race and sex for the 15 leading causes of death for the total population in 1999, United States," in *Deaths: Final Data for 1999, National Vital Statistics Reports*, v. 49, n. 8. National Center for Health Statistics, Hyattsville, MD.

Figure 1.1. Schematic of retrovirus. Centers for Disease Control and Prevention, Atlanta, GA.

Figure 1.2. Scanning electron micrograph of HTLV-III-infected T4 lymphocytes showing virus budding from the plasma membrane of the lymphocytes. Centers for Disease Control and Prevention, Atlanta, GA.

Figure 1.3. High magnification of T4 lymphocyte infected with HTLV-III. Centers for Disease Control and Prevention, Atlanta, GA.

Figure 1.4. HTLV-III/LAV-type virus in hemophilia patient who developed AIDS. Centers for Disease Control and Prevention, Atlanta, GA.

Figure 1.5. Violaceous plaques of Kaposi's sarcoma on the heel and lateral foot. Centers for Disease Control and Prevention, Atlanta, GA.

Figure 1.6. Skin biopsy of Kaposi's sarcoma. Centers for Disease Control and Prevention, Atlanta, GA.

Table 2.1. "1993 Revised Classification System for HIV Infection and Expanded Surveillance Case Definition for AIDS Among Adolescents and Adults," *Morbidity and Mortality Weekly Report*, v. 41, n. RR-17. Centers for Disease Control and Prevention, Atlanta, GA.

Table 2.2. "1993 Revised Classification System for HIV Infection and Expanded Surveillance Case Definition for AIDS Among Adolescents and Adults, *Morbidity and Mortality Weekly Report*, v. 41, n. RR-17. Centers for Disease Control and Prevention, Atlanta, GA.

Figure 2.1. "Acquired Immunodeficiency Syndrome (AIDS)—reported cases by quarter, United States, 1986-1997," in "Summary of Notifiable Diseases, United States: 1997," *Morbidity and Mortality Weekly Report*, v. 46, n. 54. Centers for Disease Control and Prevention, Atlanta, GA.

Table 2.3. "Revised Surveillance Case Definition for HIV Infection," in *CDC Guidelines for National Human Immunodeficiency Virus Case Surveillance Including Monitoring for Human Immunodeficiency Virus Infection and Acquired Immunodeficiency Syndrome, Morbidity and Mortality Weekly Report*, v. 48, n. RR-13. Centers for Disease Control and Prevention, Atlanta, GA.

Figure 2.2. "Diagram of HIV-1." Centers for Disease Control and Prevention, Atlanta, GA.

Table 3.1. "Table 1. Persons reported to be living with HIV infection and with AIDS, by area and age group, reported through December 2000," in *HIV/AIDS Surveillance Report*, v. 12, n. 2. Centers for Disease Control and Prevention, Atlanta, GA.

Table 3.2. "Table 20. Deaths in persons with AIDS, by race/ethnicity, age at death, and sex, occurring in 1998 and 1999; and cumulative totals reported through December 2000, United States," in *HIV/AIDS Surveillance Report*, v. 12, n. 2. Centers for Disease Control and Prevention, Atlanta, GA.

Table 3.3. "Table 2. AIDS cases and annual rates per 100,000 population, by area and age group, reported through December 2000, United States," in *HIV/AIDS Surveillance Report*, v. 12, n. 2. Centers for Disease Control and Prevention, Atlanta, GA.

Figure 3.1. "Figure 3. Male adult/adolescent HIV infection and AIDS cases reported in 2000, United States" and "Figure 4. Female adult/adolescent HIV infection and AIDS cases reported in 2000, United States," in *HIV/AIDS Surveillance Report*, v. 12, n. 2. Centers for Disease Control and Prevention, Atlanta, GA.

Table 3.4. "Table 4. AIDS cases and annual rates per 100,000 population, by metropolitan area and age group, reported through December 2000, United States," in *HIV/AIDS Surveillance Report*, v. 12, n. 2.

Centers for Disease Control and Prevention, Atlanta, GA.

Table 3.5. "Table 5. AIDS cases by age group, exposure category, and sex, reported through December 2000, United States," in *HIV/AIDS Surveillance Report,* v. 12, n. 2. Centers for Disease Control and Prevention, Atlanta, GA.

Table 3.6. "Table 7. AIDS cases by sex, age at diagnosis, and race/ethnicity, reported through December 2000, United States," in *HIV/AIDS Surveillance Report,* v. 12, n. 2. Centers for Disease Control and Prevention, Atlanta, GA.

Table 3.7. "Table 9. Male adult/adolescent AIDS cases by exposure category and race/ethnicity, reported through December 2000, United States," in *HIV/AIDS Surveillance Report,* v. 12, n. 2. Centers for Disease Control and Prevention, Atlanta, GA.

Table 3.8. "Table 11. Female adult/adolescent AIDS cases by exposure category and race/ethnicity, reported through December 2000, United States," in *HIV/AIDS Surveillance Report,* v. 12, n. 2. Centers for Disease Control and Prevention, Atlanta, GA.

Table 3.9. "Table 26. Estimated persons living with AIDS, by race/ethnicity and year, 1993 through 1999, United States," in *HIV/AIDS Surveillance Report,* v. 12, n. 2. Centers for Disease Control and Prevention, Atlanta, GA.

Table 3.10. "Table 18. AIDS cases and annual rates per 100,000 population, by race/ethnicity, age group, and sex, reported in 2000, United States," in *HIV/AIDS Surveillance Report,* v. 12, n. 2. Centers for Disease Control and Prevention, Atlanta, GA.

Table 3.11. "Table 15. Pediatric AIDS cases by exposure category and race/ethnicity, reported through December 2000, United States," in *HIV/AIDS Surveillance Report,* v. 12, n. 2. Centers for Disease Control and Prevention, Atlanta, GA.

Table 3.12. "Table 21. AIDS cases and deaths, by year and age group, through December 2000, United States," in *HIV/AIDS Surveillance Report,* v. 12, n. 2. Centers for Disease Control and Prevention, Atlanta, GA.

Table 3.13. "Table 30. Estimated deaths of persons with AIDS, by age group, sex, exposure category, and year of death, 1993 through 1999, United States," in *HIV/AIDS Surveillance Report,* v. 12, n. 2. Centers for Disease Control and Prevention, Atlanta, GA.

Table 4.1. "Table 12. Female adult/adolescent HIV infection cases by exposure category and race/ethnicity, reported through December 2000, from the 34 areas with confidential HIV infection reporting," in *HIV/AIDS Surveillance Report,* v. 12, n. 2. Centers for Disease Control and Prevention, Atlanta, GA.

Table 4.2. "Table 10. Male adult/adolescent HIV infection cases by exposure category and race/ethnicity, reported through December 2000, from the 34 areas with confidential HIV infection reporting," in *HIV/AIDS Surveillance Report,* v. 12, n. 2. Centers for Disease Control and Prevention, Atlanta, GA.

Table 4.3. "Table 18. AIDS cases and annual rates per 100,000 population, by race/ethnicity, age group, and sex, reported in 2000, United States," in *HIV/AIDS Surveillance Report,* v. 12, n. 2. Centers for Disease Control and Prevention, Atlanta, GA.

Table 4.4. Murphy, Sherry L., et al., "Table 8. Deaths and death rates for the 10 leading causes of death in specified age groups, by race and sex: United States, 1998," in *Deaths: Final Data for 1998, National Vital Statistics Reports,* v. 48, n. 11. National Center for Health Statistics, Hyattsville, MD.

Table 4.5. Maruschak, Laura M. "Percent of population with confirmed AIDS," in *HIV in Prisons and Jails, 1999.* U.S. Bureau of Justice Statistics, Washington DC.

Table 4.6. Maruschak, Laura M. "Table 4. Number of inmate deaths in State prisons, by cause, 1995 and 1999," in *HIV in Prisons and Jails, 1999.* U.S. Bureau of Justice Statistics, Washington DC.

Table 4.7. Maruschak, Laura M. "Table 6. Circumstances under which inmates were tested for the antibody to the human immunodeficiency virus, by jurisdiction, 1999," in *HIV in Prisons and Jails, 1999.* U.S. Bureau of Justice Statistics, Washington DC.

Table 4.8. "Table 5. AIDS cases by age group, exposure category and sex, reported through December 2000, United States," in *HIV/AIDS Surveillance Report,* v. 12, n. 2. Centers for Disease Control and Prevention, Atlanta, GA.

Table 5.1. "Table 1. Pediatric human immunodeficiency virus (HIV) classification," in *1994 Revised Classification System for HIV Infection in Children Less Than 13 Years of Age; Official Authorized Addenda: Human Immunodeficiency Virus Infection Codes and Official Guidelines for Coding and Reporting ICD-9-CM, Morbidity and Mortality Weekly Report,* v. 43, n. RR-12. Centers for Disease Control and Prevention, Atlanta, GA.

Table 5.2. "Box 1. Diagnosis of human immunodeficiency virus (HIV) infection in children," in *1994 Revised Classification System for HIV Infection in Children Less Than 13 Years of Age; Official Authorized Addenda: Human Immunodeficiency Virus Infection Codes and Official Guidelines for Coding and Reporting ICD-9-CM, Morbidity and Mortality Weekly Report,* v. 43, n. RR-12. Centers for Disease Control and Prevention, Atlanta, GA.

Table 5.3. "Table 6. HIV infection cases by age group, exposure category, and sex, reported through December 2000 from the 36 areas with confidential HIV infection reporting," in *HIV/AIDS Surveillance Report,* v. 12, n. 2. Centers for Disease Control and Prevention, Atlanta, GA.

Table 5.4. "Table 16. Pediatric HIV infection cases by exposure category and race/ethnicity, reported through December 2000, from the 36 areas with confidential HIV infection reporting," in *HIV/AIDS Surveillance Report,* v. 12, n. 2. Centers for Disease Control and Prevention, Atlanta, GA.

Figure 5.1. "Figure 5. Pediatric AIDS cases reported in 2000," in *HIV/AIDS Surveillance Report,* v. 12, n. 2. Centers for Disease Control and Prevention, Atlanta, GA.

Table 5.5. "Table 8. HIV infection cases by sex, age at diagnosis, and race/ethnicity, reported through December 2000, from the 36 areas with confidential HIV infection reporting," in *HIV/AIDS Surveillance Report,* v. 12, n. 2. Centers for Disease Control and Prevention, Atlanta, GA.

Table 5.6. "Table 14. HIV infection cases in adolescents and adults under age 25, by sex and exposure category, reported through December 2000, from the 34 areas with confidential HIV infection reporting," in *HIV/AIDS Surveillance Report,* v. 12, n. 2. Centers for Disease Control and Prevention, Atlanta, GA.

Table 6.1. Cherry, Donald K., et al. "Table 13. Number and percent of office visits with corresponding standard errors, by diagnostic and screening services ordered or provided and patient's sex: United States, 1999," in *National Ambulatory Medical Care Survey: 1999 Summary.* National Center for Health Statistics, Hyattsville, MD.

Table 6.2. Cherry, Donald K., et al. "Table 14. Number and percent of office visits with corresponding standard errors, by therapeutic and preventive services ordered or provided and patient's sex: United States, 1999," in *National Ambulatory Medical Care Survey: 1999 Summary.* National Center for Health Statistics, Hyattsville, MD.

Table 7.1. "Table 127. Federal spending for human immunodeficiency virus (HIV)-related activities, according to agency and type of activity: United States, selected fiscal years 1985-2000," in *Health, United States, 2001.* National Center for Health Statistics, Hyattsville, MD.

Table 7.2. "Ryan White CARE Act Title I Grant Awards" [Online] ftp://ftp.hrsa.gov/hab/fundinghistory.pdf [accessed December 2001]. Health Resources and Services Administration, Rockville, MD.

Table 7.3. "Ryan White CARE Act Title II Grant Awards" [Online] ftp://ftp.hrsa.gov/hab/fundinghistory/pdf [accessed December 2001]. Health Resources and Services Administration, Rockville, MD.

Figure 7.1. "Research-Based Pharmaceutical Industry R & D Spending Consistently Larger Than Entire NIH Budget (1992-2001)," in *PhRMA Annual Survey, 2001* Pharmaceutical Research & Manufacturers Of America (PhRMA). Reproduced by permission.

Table 8.1. Slome, Lee R., et al. "Characteristics of Respondents to the 1990 and 1995 Surveys," in "Physician-Assisted Suicide and Patients with Human Immunodeficiency Virus Disease," *The New England Journal of Medicine*, v. 336, n. 6, February 6, 1997. Copyright © 1997 Massachusetts Medical Society. All rights reserved. Reproduced by permission.

Table 8.2. Slome, Lee R., et al. "Responses to the Case Vignette in 1990 and 1995," in "Physician-Assisted Suicide and Patients with Human Immunodeficiency Virus Disease," *The New England Journal of Medicine*, v. 336, n. 6, February 6, 1997. Copyright © 1997 Massachusetts Medical Society. All rights reserved. Reproduced by permission.

Figure 8.1. Slome, Lee R., et al. "Distribution of the Number of Patients Assisted in Suicide, as Reported by 117 Physician Respondents to the 1995 Survey," in "Characteristics of Respondents to the 1990 and 1995 Surveys," by Lee R. Slome, et al. in "Physician-Assisted Suicide and Patients with Human Immunodeficiency Virus Disease," *The New England Journal of Medicine*, v. 336, n. 6, February 6, 1997. Copyright © 1997 Massachusetts Med-

ical Society. All rights reserved. Reproduced by permission.

Table 9.1. "Table 3. HIV infection cases by area and age group, reported through December 2000, from areas with confidential HIV infection reporting," in *HIV/AIDS Surveillance Report*, v. 12, n. 2. Centers for Disease Control and Prevention, Atlanta, GA.

Table 9.2. "Table 2. Examples of Factors that Help and Hinder CBOs to Reach their Target Populations and Deliver Interventions," in *Learning from the Community: What Community-Based Organizations Say About Factors that Affect HIV Prevention Programs*. Prepared by Conwal, Inc. for the Centers for Disease Control and Prevention, Atlanta, GA.

Table 9.3. "Table 1. Number of syringe exchange programs (SEPs), number of syringes exchanged per SEP, total number of syringes, and percentage of total number of syringes, by program size category—United States, 1998," in "Update, Syringe Exchange Programs—United States, 1998," *Morbidity and Mortality Weekly Report*, v. 50, n. 19. Centers for Disease Control and Prevention, Atlanta, GA.

Figure 10.1. "Adults and children estimated to be living with HIV/AIDS as of end 2000," in *AIDS Epidemic Update: December 2000*. Joint United Nations Programme on HIV/AIDS (UNAIDS) and World Health Organization. Reproduced by permission.

Figure 10.2. Ainsworth, Martha and Mead Over. "HIV/AIDS as a Percentage of the Infectious Disease Burden of Adults, the Developing World, 2020," in *Confronting AIDS: Public Priorities in a Global Epidemic*. The World Bank, Oxford University Press. Reproduced by permission.

Figure 10.3. Ainsworth, Martha and Mead Over. "Breakdown of Deaths from Infectious

Diseases, the Developing World, by Disease Category, 1990 and 2020 (percent)," in *Confronting AIDS: Public Priorities in a Global Epidemic*. The World Bank, Oxford University Press. Reproduced by permission.

Figure 10.4. Ainsworth, Martha and Mead Over. "The Current Impact of AIDS on Life Expectancy, Six Selected Countries, 1996," in *Confronting AIDS: Public Priorities in a Global Epidemic*. The World Bank, Oxford University Press. Reproduced by permission.

Figure 11.1. "Figure 1. Personal Concern About Becoming Infected," in *Kaiser Family Foundation National Survey of Teens on HIV/AIDS, 2000*. The Henry J. Kaiser Family Foundation, Washington, DC. This information was reprinted with permission of the Henry J. Kaiser Family Foundation of Menlo Park, California. The Kaiser Family Foundation is an independent health care philanthropy and is not associated with Kaiser Permanente or Kaiser Industries.

Figure 11.2. "Figure 2. Knowledge About Risk," in *Kaiser Family Foundation National Survey of Teens on HIV/AIDS, 2000*. The Henry J. Kaiser Family Foundation, Washington, DC. This information was reprinted with permission of the Henry J. Kaiser Family Foundation of Menlo Park, California. The Kaiser Family Foundation is an independent health care philanthropy and is not associated with Kaiser Permanente or Kaiser Industries.

Figure 11.3. "Figure 3. Teens Want to Know More," in *Kaiser Family Foundation National Survey of Teens on HIV/AIDS, 2000*. The Henry J. Kaiser Family Foundation, Washington, DC. This information was reprinted with permission of the Henry J. Kaiser Family Foundation of Menlo Park, California. The Kaiser Family Foundation is an independent health care philanthropy and is not associated with Kaiser Permanente or Kaiser Industries.

CHAPTER 1

THE NATURE OF HIV/AIDS

Acquired immune deficiency syndrome (AIDS) is the late stage of an infection caused by the human immunodeficiency virus (HIV). HIV is a retrovirus (see below) that attacks and destroys certain white blood cells, weakening the body's immune system and making it susceptible to infections and diseases that ordinarily would not be life threatening. AIDS is considered a blood-borne, sexually transmitted disease because HIV is spread through contact with blood, semen, or vaginal fluids from an infected person.

Few Americans knew of AIDS prior to 1981, when testing and reporting of the disease became mandatory, but awareness grew as the annual number of diagnosed cases and deaths steadily increased. By October 1995 the number of U.S. AIDS cases reported since 1981 reached the half-million mark. In 1995 HIV infection was the leading cause of death among persons between the ages of 25 and 44 in the United States.

By 1998, however, HIV/AIDS deaths among this age group had fallen dramatically, and HIV infection was only the fifth most common cause of death among U.S. persons between 25–44 years old. During 2000 HIV infection remained the fifth leading cause of death among persons between the ages of 25 and 44. (See Table 1.1.) Overall HIV death rates began to decline in 1996, even prior to widespread use of new and effective drug treatments such as protease inhibitors. In 1997 HIV infection was the 14th-leading cause of death overall in the United States, representing a 48 percent decline since 1996. By 1999 HIV infection no longer ranked among the 15 leading causes of death in the U.S. (See Table 1.2.)

Taken in a general sense, the decline in HIV/AIDS deaths between 1995 and 2000 seemed to indicate a positive trend for sufferers of the disease. The number of people living with HIV/AIDS during the time period increased, however, suggesting that these people would eventually need additional treatment and services. Despite the overall decline in death rates, in 1997 HIV remained a leading cause of death for African Americans between the ages of 25 and 44. By 1999 the AIDS death rate for African Americans was nearly 11 times higher than for whites. African Americans comprised 49 percent of AIDS deaths, despite representing only 13 percent of the U.S. population.

The dramatic decline in AIDS deaths between 1995 and 1997 was the result of the introduction and use of effective antiretroviral drugs that slow the progression of HIV infection. Since 1997 the rate of decline has slowed. AIDS deaths decreased only 8 percent between 1998 and 1999, compared with a 20 percent decrease between 1997 and 1998, and a 42 percent decrease between 1996 and 1997. The slowed decline in deaths may be due to a combination of several factors: patients developing resistance to drug treatments, patients inability to follow complicated drug treatment regimens, and lack of access to timely testing or treatment. According to the Centers for Disease Control (CDC), through December 2000, 775,299 people in the U.S. were reported to have contracted AIDS, and 448,060 of these people have died. The CDC estimates about 900,000 people in the United States are living with HIV, and approximately 40,000 people become infected every year.

Researchers for the Joint United Nations Programme on HIV/AIDS (UNAIDS) and the World Health Organization (WHO) report that AIDS has become a global epidemic that exceeds predictions made ten years ago by 50 percent. According to the December 2000 *AIDS Epidemic Update*, 36.1 million people worldwide are living with HIV/AIDS. The organization estimates that in 2000, 5.3 million people were newly infected and 3 million people worldwide died of AIDS. The countries of Sub-Saharan Africa continued to have the world's highest annual rates of HIV infection in 2000. In South Africa, 4 million people—nearly 10 percent of that nation's population—were estimated to be HIV-positive.

TABLE 1.1

Deaths and death rates for the 10 leading causes of death in specified age groups, preliminary 2000

[Data are based on a continuous file of records received from the states. Rates per 100,000 population in specified group. Figures are based on weighted data rounded to the nearest individual, so categories may not add to totals.]

Rank [1]	Cause of death and age (Based on the Tenth Revision, International Classification of Diseases, 1992)	Number	Rate
	15-24 years		
...	All causes	30,959	80.7
1	Accidents (unintentional injuries) (V01-X59,Y85-Y86)	13,616	35.5
...	Motor vehicle accidents (V02-V04,V09.0,V09.2,V12-V14,V19.0-V19.2,V19.4-V19.6,V20-V79,V80.3-V80.5, V81.1,V82.0-V82.1,V83-V86,V87.0-V87.8,V88.0-V88.8,V89.0,V89.2)	10,357	27.0
...	All other accidents (V01,V05-V06,V09.1,V09.3-V09.9,V10-V11,V15-V18,V19.3,V19.8-V19.9,V80.0-V80.2, V80.6-V80.9,V81.2-V81.9,V82.2-V82.9,V87.9,V88.9,V89.1,V89.3,V89.9,V90-V99,W00-X59,Y85,Y86)	3,259	8.5
2	Assault (homicide) (X85-Y09,Y87.1)	4,796	12.5
3	Intentional self-harm (suicide) (X60-X84,Y87.0)	3,877	10.1
4	Malignant neoplasms (C00-C97)	1,668	4.3
5	Diseases of heart (I00-I09,I11,I13,I20-I51)	931	2.4
6	Congenital malformations, deformations and chromosomal abnormalities (Q00-Q99)	425	1.1
7	Cerebrovascular diseases (I60-I69)	193	0.5
8	Influenza and pneumonia (J10-J18)	188	0.5
9	Chronic lower respiratory diseases (J40-J47)	180	0.5
10	Human immunodeficiency virus (HIV) disease (B20-B24)	178	0.5
...	All other causes (Residual)	4,907	12.8
	25-44 years		
...	All causes	128,779	156.4
1	Accidents (unintentional injuries) (V01-X59,Y85-Y86)	24,817	30.1
...	Motor vehicle accidents (V02-V04,V09.0,V09.2,V12-V14,V19.0-V19.2,V19.4-V19.6,V20-V79,V80.3-V80.5, V81.0-V81.1,V82.0-V82.1,V83-V86,V87.0-V87.8,V88.0-V88.8,V89.0,V89.2)	13,261	16.1
...	All other accidents (V01,V05-V06,V09.1,V09.3-V09.9,V10-V11,V15-V18,V19.3,V19.8-V19.9,V80.0-V80.2, V80.6-V80.9,V81.2-V81.9,V82.2-V82.9,V87.9,V88.9,V89.1,V89.3,V89.9,V90-V99,W00-X59,Y85,Y86)	11,556	14.0
2	Malignant neoplasms (C00-C97)	20,200	24.5
3	Diseases of heart (I00-I09,I11,I13,I20-I51)	15,267	18.5
4	Intentional self-harm (suicide) (X60-X84,Y87.0)	10,884	13.2
5	Human immunodeficiency virus (HIV) disease (B20-B24)	8,302	10.1
6	Assault (homicide) (X85-Y09,Y87.1)	7,156	8.7
7	Chronic liver disease and cirrhosis (K70,K73-K74)	3,644	4.4
8	Cerebrovascular diseases (I60-I69)	3,122	3.8
9	Diabetes mellitus (E10-E14)	2,416	2.9
10	Influenza and pneumonia (J10-J18)	1,437	1.7
...	All other causes (Residual)	31,534	38.3
	45-64 years		
...	All causes	399,008	652.8
1	Malignant neoplasms (C00-C97)	136,363	223.1
2	Diseases of heart (I00-I09,I11,I13,I20-I51)	97,334	159.2
3	Accidents (unintentional injuries) (V01-X59,Y85-Y86)	18,252	29.9
...	Motor vehicle accidents (V02-V04,V09.0,V09.2,V12-V14,V19.0-V19.2,V19.4-V19.6,V20-V79,V80.3-V80.5, V81.0-V81.1,V82.0-V82.1,V83-V86,V87.0-V87.8,V88.0-V88.8,V89.0,V89.2)	8,483	13.9
...	All other accidents (V01,V05-V06,V09.1,V09.3-V09.9,V10-V11,V15-V18,V19.3,V19.8-V19.9,V80.0-V80.2, V80.6-V80.9,V81.2-V81.9,V82.2-V82.9,V87.9,V88.9,V89.1,V89.3,V89.9,V90-V99,W00-X59,Y85,Y86)	9,769	16.0
4	Cerebrovascular diseases (I60-I69)	15,735	25.7
5	Chronic lower respiratory diseases (J40-J47)	14,086	23.0
6	Diabetes mellitus (E10-E14)	13,958	22.8
7	Chronic liver disease and cirrhosis (K70,K73-K74)	12,206	20.0
8	Intentional self-harm (suicide) (X60-X84,Y87.0)	8,052	13.2
9	Human immunodeficiency virus (HIV) disease (B20-B24)	5,336	8.7
10	Nephritis, nephrotic syndrome and nephrosis (N00-N07,N17-N19,N25-N27)	4,821	7.9
...	All other causes (Residual)	72,865	119.2

NOTE: Data are subject to sampling and/or random variation.
... Category not applicable.
[1]Rank based on number of deaths.

SOURCE: Adapted from Arialdi M. Minino and Betty L. Smith, "Table 7. Deaths and death rates for the 10 leading causes of death in specified age groups: United States, preliminary 2000," in "Deaths: Preliminary Data for 2000," *National Vital Statistics Reports*, vol. 49, no. 12, National Center for Health Statistics, Hyattsville, MD, October 9, 2001

THE HUMAN IMMUNODEFICIENCY VIRUS

A virus is a tiny infectious agent composed of genes surrounded by a protective coating. Viruses are parasites that must invade other cells in order to reproduce. The invaded cells serve as their own death chambers because the virus reproduces so proficiently that the cells are destroyed and the host (in the case of HIV, a human) becomes diseased. Common colds, influenza (flu), and some forms of pneumonia are caused by viruses.

HIV belongs to a group of viruses known as retroviruses, which have a special enzyme that reverses the

TABLE 1.2

Fifteen leading causes of death for the total population, 1999

[Death rates on an annual basis per 100,000 population; age-adjusted rates per 100,000 U.S. standard population based on year 2000 standard]

Rank[1]	Cause of death (Based on the *Tenth Revision International Classification of Diseases, 1992*)	Number	Percent of total deaths	1999 crude death rate	Age-adjusted death rate — 1999	Percent change[2] 1998 to 1999	Ratio — Male to female	Ratio — Black to white	Ratio — Hispanic to white non-Hispanic
...	All causes	2,391,399	100.0	877.0	881.9	0.7	1.4	1.3	0.7
1	Diseases of heart	I00–I09,I11,I13,I51 725,192	30.3	265.9	267.8	−0.3	1.5	1.3	0.7
2	Malignant neoplasms	C00–C97 549,838	23.0	201.6	202.7	−0.5	1.5	1.3	0.6
3	Cerebrovascular diseases	I60–I69 167,366	7.0	61.4	61.8	−1.9	1.0	1.4	0.7
4	Chronic lower respiratory diseases	J40–J47 124,181	5.2	45.5	45.8	4.1	1.5	0.7	0.4
5	Accidents (unintentional injuries)	V01–X59,Y85–Y86 97,860	4.1	35.9	35.9	−0.6	2.2	1.1	0.9
6	Diabetes mellitus	E10–E14 68,399	2.9	25.1	25.2	3.3	1.2	2.2	1.5
7	Influenza and pneumonia	J10–J18 63,730	2.7	23.4	23.6	−2.5	1.3	1.1	0.7
8	Alzheimer's disease	G30 44,536	1.9	16.3	16.5	[3]23.1	0.8	0.7	0.4
9	Nephritis, nephrotic syndrome and nephrosis	N00–N07,N17–N19,N25–N27 35,525	1.5	13.0	13.1	[3]8.3	1.4	2.5	0.9
10	Septicemia	A40–A41 30,680	1.3	11.3	11.3	6.6	1.2	2.5	0.8
11	Intentional self-harm (suicide)	X60–X84,Y87.0 29,199	1.2	10.7	10.7	−5.3	4.4	0.5	0.5
12	Chronic liver disease and cirrhosis	K70,K73–K74 26,259	1.1	9.6	9.7	−1.0	2.2	1.1	1.7
13	Essential (primary) hypertension and hypertensive renal disease	I10,I12 16,968	0.7	6.2	6.3	5.0	1.0	3.0	1.0
14	Assault (homicide)	X85–Y09,Y87.1 16,889	0.7	6.2	6.2	−4.6	3.2	5.4	2.9
15	Aortic aneurysm and dissection	I71 15,807	0.7	5.8	5.8	−4.9	2.3	0.8	0.4
...	All other causes	Residual 378,970	15.8	139.0	...	...	...	...	...

– Quantity zero.
... Category not applicable.
[1] Rank based on number of deaths.
[2] Percent change is based on a comparison of the 1999 age-adjusted death rate with the 1998 comparability-modified, age-adjusted death rate.
[3] Percent change is not reliable because of problems in measuring comparability.

SOURCE: "Table C. Percent of total deaths, death rates, age-adjusted death rates for 1999, percent change in age-adjusted death rates from 1998 to 1999 and ratio of age-adjusted death rates by race and sex for the 15 leading causes of death for the total population in 1999, United States," in *Deaths: Final Data for 1999,* National Vital Statistics Report, vol. 49, no. 8, National Center for Health Statistics, Hyattsville, MD, September 21, 2001

usual pattern of translating the genetic message. (See Figure 1.1.) In animals, genes are stored in DNA. This DNA serves as a template from which RNA is transcribed. The RNA is then translated into protein. Retroviruses have their genes stored in RNA. Instead of transcribing from DNA (deoxyribonucleic acid, the chemical composition of genes in living cells) to RNA (ribonucleic acid, a chemical necessary for cell function), retroviruses transcribe in reverse. After HIV infects a human cell, the HIV RNA is reverse transcribed into DNA. This viral DNA is then integrated into the host's DNA and is eventually used to make additional copies of HIV.

Retroviruses had been found in some animals, but the first human retroviruses, human T cell leukemia virus (HTLV-I) and the very closely related human T cell lymphotropic virus (HTLV-II), were discovered in 1980 by Dr. Robert Gallo and his colleagues at the U.S. National Cancer Institute (NCI). This breakthrough provided the groundwork for the discovery of the virus that would eventually be known as HIV.

Identifying the Virus

In September 1983 Dr. Luc Montagnier and researchers at the Pasteur Institute in Paris, France, isolated and identi-fied a retrovirus that they named lymphadenopathy-associated virus (LAV). Eight months later Dr. Gallo's group at NCI isolated the same virus in AIDS patients, which they called HTLV-III. LAV and HTLV-III were found to be identical and are now referred to as HIV. A conflict arose about which researcher should be credited with the discovery, and in 1991, in an intense, politically charged atmosphere, Dr. Gallo dropped his claim to the discovery of HIV.

The Origins of the Virus

It has long been speculated that HIV evolved from a retrovirus that infected monkeys called simian immunodeficiency virus (SIV). The theory is that HIV evolved from human infection with monkey viruses that mutated inside human's bodies.

In 1982 Isao Miyoshi of Kochi University identified an HTLV-related virus in the Japanese macaque monkey. Genetically similar to HTLV, it was designated as the simian T-lymphotropic virus (STLV). Further studies found STLV present in both Asian and African Old World monkeys and apes with an infection rate ranging from 1 to 40 percent.

Dr. Max Essex and Dr. Phyllis T. Kanki of the Harvard School of Public Health discovered that the simian

FIGURE 1.1

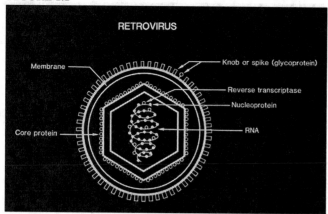

Schematic of a retrovirus. *Centers for Disease Control and Prevention*

virus found in the African chimpanzee and the African green monkey was more homologous (related in primitive origin) to the human virus than the simian virus in the Asian macaque. This discovery demonstrated the likely significance of African STLV in the origin and evolution of human HTLV.

In 1986 scientists at the Pasteur Institute discovered a new AIDS-causing virus in West Africans. They labeled the virus HIV-2, a milder form of HIV that differs in molecular structure from the earlier HIV-1 and seems to be closely related to a virus that causes AIDS in macaque monkeys. The CDC estimates that as of 1998, 79 people in the United States had been infected with HIV-2. (Unless otherwise specified, the term HIV in this publication refers to HIV-1.)

Along with the majority of investigators, Dr. Gallo and Dr. Montagnier believe the virus has been present in Central Africa and other regions for some time. The rural nature of these societies and the limited access to the outside world by those infected with the virus may have contained HIV for many decades. Once persons in Central Africa began migrating to urban areas where sexual practices were not as strict as those in tribal life, HIV spread more easily and quickly. Within a comparatively short time, the once rare and remote disease was spread by HIV-infected people who traveled around the world.

ATTACKING THE IMMUNE SYSTEM

To learn how HIV first attacks healthy cells while evading attack by the immune system, it is important to understand the complex structure of HIV and how normal white blood cells work.

Healthy White Blood Cells at Work

White blood cells are major components of the complicated, coordinated system of organs and cells that make up the human immune system. These cells and organs work together to prevent invasion by foreign substances. The five types of white blood cells are macrophages (scavenger cells of the immune system), T4 or helper T cells, T8 or killer T cells, plasma B cells, and memory B cells. T and B cells constitute a class of white blood cells called lymphocytes that bear the major responsibility for carrying out immune system activities.

Each type of white blood cell has a specific function. The macrophage, which begins as a smaller monocyte (single cell), readies the T4 cells to respond to particular invaders such as viruses. At the time of attack, the macrophage, sometimes referred to as the vacuum cleaner of the immune system, swallows the virus, leaving a portion displayed so that the T4 cell can make contact. The macrophage also stimulates production of thousands of T4 cells, all programmed to battle the invader.

When T4 lymphocytes attack an invading virus, they also send out chemical messages that cause the multiplication of B cells and T8 "killer cells," which, with the help of some T4 cells, destroy the infected cell. Other T4 cells, which are not actively involved in destroying the infected cells, send chemical messages to B cells, causing them to reproduce and divide into groups of either plasma cells or memory cells. Plasma cells make antibodies that cripple the invading virus, while memory cells increase the immune response in the event that the invader ever attacks again.

HIV's Molecular Structure

HIV, which has seven types of genes, is far more complex than most other retroviruses, which have only three or four genes. Scientists believe that these genes direct the production of proteins that make up parts of the virus and regulate its reproduction. The HIV core contains genes that are protected by a protein shell, while the entire virus is surrounded by a fatty membrane dotted with glycoproteins (proteins with sugar units attached), adding to its protection. Figures 1.2 through 1.4 show microscopic views of HIV in various stages of development.

Once HIV enters the human body, it primarily attacks a subset of immune cells that contains a molecule called CD4. In particular, the virus attaches itself to two types of CD4-containing cells: CD4+ T cells and, to a lesser extent, macrophages.

A New Discovery

In 1995 researchers at Oxford University in England posited that HIV, by subtle mutation, actually defuses the killer cells that are supposed to destroy virus-stricken cells. When the Oxford researchers isolated HIV from patients, they found that the viruses had undergone a mutation, or change, in their genetic structure. When killer T cells approached cells infected with the mutated virus, the T cells failed to kill the stricken cells, perhaps because they

FIGURE 1.2

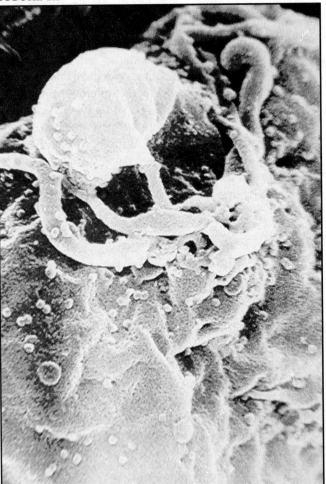

A scanning electron micrograph of HTLV-III-infected T4 lymphocytes, showing the virus budding from the plasma membrane of the lymphocytes. *Centers for Disease Control and Prevention*

FIGURE 1.3

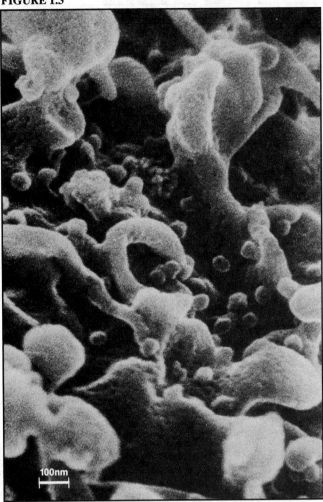

High magnification view of a T4 lymphocyte infected with HTLV-III. *Centers for Disease Control and Prevention*

no longer recognized them. The T cells were in fact unable to kill even cells infected with the original, unmutated virus. The mutations not only allowed the altered strains to multiply, but also allowed unaltered strains to flourish.

ANOTHER THEORY: "FRIENDLY FIRE." Not all researchers agree. Some believe that other cells in the immune system attack and kill CD4-containing cells in what has been termed an "autoimmune response." Some CD4-containing cells that have not been invaded by the virus, but display fragments of it, become targets for other cells—in addition to the killer cells—which see the infected cells as a camouflaged virus and kill them. In addition, HIV-infected cells may send out protein signals that weaken or destroy other healthy cells in the immune system.

HIV then exhibits various behaviors, depending on the kind of cell it has invaded and how the cell behaves. In T cells the virus can remain dormant for 2–20 years, hidden from the immune system. When the cells are stimulated, however, the viral genes that have been incorporated into the DNA of the T4 cells can duplicate copies of the virus that then break free of the T4 cells and attack other cells. Once a T4 cell has been infected, it cannot respond adequately and may reproduce as few as 10 cells instead of the 1,000 or more needed to fight the invader. When these cells do encounter the invader, the virus inside them reproduces and the cells are destroyed. To make the situation even worse, HIV reproduces itself at a rate far greater than any other known virus. The T4 cells essentially become factories for the invading enemy soldiers, ultimately producing them in overwhelming numbers.

Because of the many ways HIV attacks the immune system and its ability to mutate, researchers believe it will be very difficult to develop an effective vaccine. Testing a vaccine is also difficult, since people cannot be deliberately contaminated with HIV in order to ascertain the effectiveness of a vaccine.

The Attack

The immune system is unable to produce sufficient antibodies to fight off the complex human immunodeficiency

FIGURE 1.4

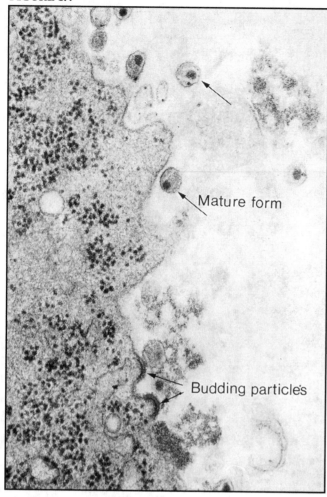

Mature form

Budding particles

The HTLV-III/LAV-type virus, found in a hemophilia patient who developed AIDS. *Centers for Disease Control and Prevention*

virus. The battle between HIV and the immune system begins when the virus slips into the bloodstream via a CD4 receptor enzyme on a T4 cell, to which it preferentially attaches itself. A CD4 receptor alone, however, is not enough to cause infection, and for years scientists searched for some other protein on the cell surface that HIV can exploit to gain entry.

This protein was discovered in May 1996 by a team of scientists at the National Institute of Allergy and Infectious Diseases (NIAID) in Bethesda, Maryland. The scientists named the protein "fusin" because it helps the virus fuse with a healthy cell membrane and inject genetic material into the cell. The CD4-containing cell signals to killer T cells that it is infected by displaying fragments of HIV proteins on its surface. This triggers the killer cells to spring into action, multiplying and seeking out the infected CD4-containing cells in order to pierce them open and destroy them.

CONFIRMING A HIDING PLACE

Typically an HIV infection begins with a sudden, flu-like illness. Shortly after this first episode, the virus virtu-

ally disappears and symptoms may not materialize for as long as 20 years. Over time, the immune system eventually collapses and the virus appears in ever-increasing amounts of CD4-containing cells floating free in the patients' blood. While previous studies had focused on the presence of the virus in the blood, two independently conducted studies in 1993 confirmed suspicions long held by scientists that HIV hides in a patient's lymph nodes and similar tissue during the quiescent (first or early) stage of infection. In March 1993 Dr. Anthony S. Fauci and his colleagues from NIAID and Dr. Ashley T. Haase and his colleagues from the University of Minnesota published papers describing the hiding places of HIV (*Science*, Vol. 262, November 12, 1993, pp. 110, 111–18).

Searching for an Active Virus

Dr. Fauci's research focused on the search for the virus in the blood and lymphoid tissue (the lymph nodes, spleen, tonsils, and adenoids) of 12 infected patients in various stages of HIV infection. Initially the virus is concentrated almost entirely in the lymphoid tissues. Particles of the virus, coated with antibodies, adhere to the follicular dendritic cells, a group of filtering cells that trap foreign material. CD4-containing cells nearby see the trapped material and are stimulated to attack the invaders. The stronger virus counterattacks and reproduces itself on some of these CD4-containing cells. Dr. Fauci believes that the virus infiltrates the lymph nodes within weeks of the initial infection.

After this infiltration, over an extended period of time (perhaps as long as 20 years) the immune system begins to dramatically decline. During this decline the follicular dendritic cells also begin to deteriorate and the quantity of HIV in the CD4-containing cells floating free in the blood significantly increases. In the final stage of the disease there is an almost complete dissolution of the follicular dendritic cell network. At this point, the amount of HIV in the blood and in the CD4-containing cells has grown to equal the amount in the lymph nodes.

NOT JUST THE IMMUNE SYSTEM

For some time, scientists and researchers believed HIV attacked and affected only the immune system. Many early AIDS cases were not counted because of the narrower definitions of AIDS that existed before 1993. After 1993 clear evidence showed that the free virus (not attached to any other cells) could appear in the fluid surrounding the brain and the spinal cord and in the bloodstream. HIV can be found not only in T4 lymphocytes, but also in other immune system cells, as well as in cells in the nervous system, intestine, and bone marrow.

Researchers at the CDC proposed another reason why HIV infections are so difficult to eliminate and why the immune system appears to be so susceptible to them. Their research showed that HIV could infect and grow in very immature bone marrow cells, offering no clues about what the mature HIV-infected cells would become. The virus self-reproduces without revealing itself to the immune system, which under normal circumstances would destroy it. By developing in immature bone marrow cells, a great quantity of virus can be produced before the body ever attempts to resist it.

As they mature the cells change, becoming infected monocytes and macrophages that may not only fail to fight infections, but also may spread the virus to other immune system cells. Infected marrow cells may seed the virus into other parts of the body, including the brain. The infected cells that develop in the marrow are carried through the bloodstream to the rest of the body.

SEARCHING FOR ANSWERS

Scientists have long been puzzled by the fact that AIDS is virtually always fatal, although relatively small amounts of the virus are found in patients. Theories abound as to exactly how the virus acts to kill the cells, since it is normally not the nature of retroviruses to kill all the cells in the host. Although HIV is considered a slow virus, some AIDS activity is fast-paced and may be caused by the presence of a mycoplasma (a class of bacteria that lack cell walls and may cause disease) infection.

Restoring Immune Response

In December 1993 the NCI reported that the immune function had been restored to HIV-infected cells grown in a laboratory by adding interleukin-12 (IL-12), a member of a group of natural blood proteins called cytokines that were discovered in 1991 by scientists at the Wistar Institute in Philadelphia, Pennsylvania, and Hoffman-LaRoche, Inc., in Nutley, New Jersey. The Food and Drug Administration (FDA) halted human testing of IL-12 in June 1995 when two patients died. After testing the protein on animals, researchers concluded that the problem was not in IL-12 itself, but in the timing of the doses. Consequently, human testing resumed in November 1995.

In December 1995 a new class of drugs called protease inhibitors received FDA approval. These drugs block the ability of HIV to mature and to infect new cells by suppressing a protein enzyme of the virus, protease, which is crucial to the life cycle of HIV. If protease inhibitors can block the spread of HIV in the immune system, then AIDS will not develop. Though patients may be HIV-positive the rest of their lives, they may never die from HIV infection.

Theories of HIV/AIDS Progression

Even after more than two decades of research, experts in the study of HIV still do not agree on the pathogenesis (the origination and development) of AIDS. Most concur, however, that the period between HIV infection and the symptomatic stage of AIDS averages from about 2 to 11 years, but can last as long as 20 years. Further, a very small proportion of individuals, between 5 and 10 percent of all HIV-infected persons, do not appear to develop AIDS. Called "long-term nonprogressors," these individuals are believed to have genetic and immune response characteristics that slow, or may even halt, the course of disease progression.

Martin A. Nowak, in the *Journal of Acquired Immune Deficiency Syndrome and Human Retrovirology* ("AIDS Pathogenesis: From Models to Viral Dynamics in Patients," December 1995), noted that after HIV infection, the immune system regenerates cells only up to a certain point, which would explain a gradual progression to AIDS. The early regulatory functions of the immune system limit viral replication until a certain threshold is reached. When the number of different viral mutants becomes too large, the regulatory system is overwhelmed and shuts down, opening the door to opportunistic infections and eventual total decline.

When the total CD4+ T cell count falls from the normal 800–1,000 per cubic millimeters of blood to 200 per cubic millimeters, the rate of decline speeds up and the HIV-positive patient becomes prone to the opportunistic infections and other illnesses that are characteristic of AIDS. In searching for an antiretroviral therapy, researchers found that rather than boosting the CD4+ T cell count, interruption of the viral replication may be the way to reverse immune deficiency in HIV infection, though the nature of a reversing mechanism remains unknown.

SOME INCONSISTENCIES WITH CURRENT THEORIES. Most scientists agree that there are major gaps and inconsistencies in the knowledge of how HIV causes AIDS. One inconsistency deals with the infection and killing of the helper T cells. Initially, researchers thought that the main tactic of HIV was to infect and destroy the T cells. As these cells died, the numerical strength of the helper T cell force must be depleted, causing the immune deficiency associated with persons with AIDS.

Other scientists, however, consider this theory too simplistic, since so few T cells—no more than 1 infected cell in 500—are infected. Another inconsistency involves the observation that the rapid decline in the number of T cells comes relatively late in the infection, even though there are clear indications that the immune system has been impaired much earlier.

CIGARETTES AND ALCOHOL SPEED DEVELOPMENT OF AIDS. Experts believe that cigarette and alcohol use accelerate the development of AIDS symptoms. They counsel HIV-positive patients to abandon smoking and drinking alcohol because research shows that the use of these products suppresses immune response.

FIGURE 1.5

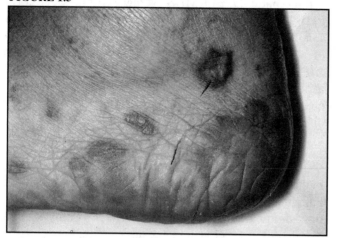

Violaceous plaques of Kaposi's sarcoma on the heel and lateral foot. *Centers for Disease Control and Prevention*

FIGURE 1.6

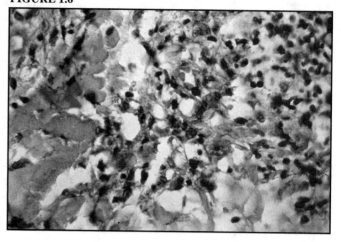

A skin biopsy of Kaposi's sarcoma. *Centers for Disease Control and Prevention*

OPPORTUNISTIC INFECTIONS

Once HIV has destroyed the immune system, the body can no longer protect itself against bacterial, fungal, protozoal, and other viral agents that take advantage of the compromised condition, causing opportunistic infections (OIs). Opportunistic infections are illnesses caused by organisms that normally would not harm a healthy person. Because the patient is considered to have AIDS if at least one opportunistic infection appears, OIs are also referred to as "AIDS-defining events," though OIs are not the only AIDS-defining events.

In 1997 the leading OI for persons in the United States suffering from HIV/AIDS was *Pneumocystis carinii* pneumonia (PCP), a lung disease caused by a fungus and, prior to the discovery of HIV/AIDS, found almost exclusively in cancer and transplant patients with weakened immune systems. PCP has been declining since 1987, most likely due to better treatment and earlier diagnosis. Esophageal candidiasis, an infection of the esophagus, and extrapulmonary cryptococcosis, a systemic fungus that enters the body through the lungs and may invade any organ of the body, are also OIs frequently diagnosed in AIDS patients.

Other illnesses such as Burkitt's lymphoma, invasive cervical cancer, and primary brain lymphoma are also considered AIDS-defining events. Wasting syndrome (which includes sudden weight loss and lethargy) is another illness that may be considered an AIDS-defining event. Other examples of AIDS-defining events include diagnosis of *Mycobacterium avium complex (MAC)*, a serious bacterial infection that may occur in one part of the body such as the liver, bone marrow, and spleen or spread throughout the body; cytomegalovirus disease (CMV), a member of the herpesvirus group; Kaposi's sarcoma, a once-rare cancer of the blood vessel walls that causes conspicuous purple lesions on the skin (see Figure 1.5 and Figure 1.6); and toxoplasmic encephalitis, an inflammation of the brain. Patients may experience more than one OI or AIDS-defining event.

HIV and Tuberculosis

Tuberculosis (TB), a communicable disease caused by the bacterium *Mycobacterium tuberculosis*, is occurring with increasing frequency among persons infected with HIV. HIV infection has in fact become one of the strongest known risk factors for the progression of TB from infection to disease. A 1996 report from the Conference on Retroviruses and Opportunistic Infections concluded that the decline in CD4+ T cells is greater in HIV-infected patients who develop TB than in those who remain free of the disease. In some geographic areas as many as 58 percent of persons diagnosed with TB were also HIV-positive. Of the many diseases associated with HIV infection, TB is one of the few that is transmissible, treatable, and preventable.

TB is spread from person to person through the inhalation of airborne particles containing *M. tuberculosis*. The particles, called droplet nuclei, are produced when a person with infectious TB of the lung or larynx forcefully exhales, such as when coughing, sneezing, speaking, or singing. These infectious particles remain suspended in the air and may be inhaled by someone sharing the same air. Risk of transmission is increased where ventilation is poor and when susceptible persons share air for prolonged periods with a person who has untreated pulmonary TB.

Most TB (approximately 85 percent) occurs in the lungs and is termed pulmonary TB. The disease may occur at any site of the body, however, such as the larynx, the lymph nodes, the brain, the kidneys, or the bones; such cases are termed extrapulmonary TB. With the exception of laryngeal TB, persons with extrapulmonary

TB are usually not considered infectious to others. It is important to note that, as mentioned earlier in this chapter, HIV is a blood-borne infection and cannot be spread through air. An HIV-positive person who has TB can spread TB nuclei through the air, but not HIV.

TB does not develop in everyone who is infected with the bacteria. In the United States about 90 percent of infected persons remain infected for life, yet never develop symptoms of TB. However, in about 5 percent of persons, the disease develops in the first or second year after infection, and in another 5 percent, it develops later in life. The risk that TB will develop in people infected with TB and HIV is about 8 percent per year. In contrast, the risk that it will develop in those infected only with TB is 5–10 percent within their entire lifetime.

HIV and Cancer

People with AIDS are susceptible to cancer. Some malignant tumors, such as Kaposi's sarcoma and cancers of the lymph system, have been common among AIDS patients since the disease was first discovered in 1981. Now, however, doctors and researchers are beginning to find that as HIV/AIDS patients live longer, certain forms of cancer are becoming more prevalent among them. Most AIDS-related cancers are cancers believed to be caused by viruses. These cancers are more common among HIV-infected persons because HIV suppresses the immune system, enabling cancer-causing viruses to attack more successfully. These cancers include non-Hodgkin's lymphoma (found in lymph tissues) and primary lymphoma of the brain. People infected with HIV are also at greater risk of myeloma (malignant tumors of the bone marrow), brain tumors, testicular cancers, and leukemia.

In June 1998 the National Cancer Institute held its second international meeting devoted to HIV/AIDS and cancer. The primary focus of the meeting was to determine the impact of the new anti-HIV drugs on AIDS-related cancers. Researchers reported a decline in Kaposi's sarcoma and primary lymphoma of the brain since newer anti-HIV combination drug therapies have become available. One possible explanation for the decline may be that the combination drug therapies enable the body to recover partial immunity, which in turn controls the cancer. While the decline appears real, investigators believe it is too early to accept these findings until a longer-term follow-up has been completed.

CHAPTER 2
DEFINITION, SYMPTOMS, AND TRANSMITTAL

A DEFINITION OF AIDS

The Centers for Disease Control and Prevention (CDC) in Atlanta, Georgia, a branch of the U.S. Public Health Service, is the federal government's clearinghouse, research center, and monitoring agency for all infectious diseases, including HIV/AIDS. The CDC tracks and then notifies health officials nationwide of diseases in the United States. It defines AIDS as a specific group of diseases or conditions that are indicative of severe immunosuppression related to infection with the human immunodeficiency virus (HIV). The CDC first outlined a surveillance (constant observation of a process) case definition in 1982, then revised it in 1983, 1985, 1987, 1993, and again in 2000 as knowledge about HIV infection increased and additional severe and common symptoms were included in the definitions. The January 1, 1993, definition emphasized the clinical importance of the CD4+ T cell count and included the addition of three clinical conditions.

THE 1993 CLASSIFICATION REVISION AND EXPANDED SURVEILLANCE CASE DEFINITION

In 1991 the CDC released a draft of the document that would become the *1993 Revised Classification for HIV Infection and Expanded AIDS Surveillance Case Definition for Adolescents and Adults*. Many women, their physicians, and attorneys had strongly advocated the inclusion of diseases such as pelvic inflammatory disease and vaginal candidiasis as conditions indicating a progression to AIDS, so that women infected with HIV would be included in the revised definition. Advocates cautioned that if the CDC omitted such inclusive criteria, many women would be denied access to disability benefits, necessary treatment, and education.

Reasons for Expanding the Case Definition

The CDC reported three reasons for expanding the AIDS surveillance case definitions:

1. **To be consistent with standards of medical care for HIV-infected persons.** The addition of a measurement for severe immunosuppression (a CD4+ T lymphocyte count of 200 per cubic millimeter or less than 14 percent of total lymphocytes) is consistent with the standard used to determine clinical and therapeutic treatment of HIV-infected persons. (It is important to note that a person can be HIV-infected and not have AIDS.) At present, some clinicians recommend a conservative approach—that all persons with a count of 500 CD4+ T cells per cubic millimeter or less be given antiretroviral therapy. Others advocate more aggressive treatment; these clinicians begin antiretroviral therapy as soon as the diagnosis of HIV infection is made. Prophylaxis (prevention treatment) against *Pneumocystis carinii* pneumonia (PCP), the most common serious opportunistic infection (OI) should be started on patients with a count of 200 CD4+ T cells per cubic millimeter or less.

2. **To include persons with conditions of major public health importance in the HIV epidemic.** The inclusion of HIV-infected persons with low CD4+ T cell counts allows the HIV/AIDS surveillance to reflect more accurately the number of persons who have severe immunosuppression. These persons are in greatest need of close medical follow-up and at greatest risk for many or all of the severe HIV-related illnesses. The addition of three clinical conditions—pulmonary TB, recurrent pneumonia, and invasive cervical cancer—to the 23 already accepted conditions of AIDS surveillance criteria indicates the documented or potential importance of these diseases in the HIV epidemic. Two of these conditions, pulmonary TB and cervical cancer, are preventable with appropriate screening tests and proper follow-up. The third condition, recurrent pneumonia, was included to show the importance of pulmonary infections in the causes of HIV-related diseases and deaths.

TABLE 2.1

1993 revised classification system for HIV infection and expanded AIDS surveillance case definition for AIDS among adolescents and adults[1]

CD4+ T-cell categories	Clinical categories		
	(A) Asymptomatic, acute (primary) HIV or PGL[2]	(B) Symptomatic, not (A) or (C) conditions	(C) AIDS-indicator conditions
(1) ≥500/μL	A1	B1	C1
(2) 200–499/μL	A2	B2	C2
(3) <200/μL AIDS-indicator T-cell count	A3	B3	C3

[1] The shaded cells illustrate the expanded AIDS surveillance case definition. Persons with AIDS-indicator conditions (Category C) as well as those with CD4+ T-lymphocyte counts <200/μL (Categories A3 or B3) will be reportable as AIDS cases in the United States and Territories, effective January 1, 1993.

[2] PGL = persistent generalized lymphadenopathy. Clinical Category A includes acute (primary) HIV infection.

SOURCE: "1993 Revised Classification System for HIV Infection and Expanded Surveillance Case Definition for AIDS Among Adolescents and Adults," *Morbidity and Mortality Weekly Report*, vol. 41, no. RR-17, December 18, 1992

3. **To simplify the AIDS case-reporting process.** The CDC tried to simplify the AIDS case-reporting process by allowing clinicians to report HIV-infected persons on the basis of CD4+ T cell counts. Limited staff at outpatient clinics and the increasing proportion of AIDS cases necessitated the use of a simplified AIDS surveillance case definition.

New Definition and Classification—Tied to CD4+ Cells

One of the major obstacles in defining AIDS has been that it is not a single disease but several diseases making up a syndrome. Newer preventive treatments delay the onset of many diseases such as PCP, which in the past helped to define AIDS. In order to obtain a more realistic picture of the number of AIDS cases, the new classification system emphasized the importance of the CD4+ or helper T cell count.

Based on this, the 1993 definition included all HIV-infected persons with a CD4+ T cell count of less than 200 per cubic millimeter or whose CD4+ T cell count is less than 14 percent of total lymphocytes. In essence, most persons with very low T4 counts would be defined as having AIDS. As shown in Table 2.1, the 1993 classification system was based on three ranges of CD4+ T cell counts and three clinical categories, represented by a combination of nine categories. Persons with AIDS-indicator conditions (Category C) or those with CD4+ T cell counts of less than 200 per cubic millimeter meet the immunologic criteria for the AIDS surveillance case definition.

Table 2.2 gives a more detailed description of Categories A and B, as well as the clinical conditions listed in Category C. Note that for classification purposes, once a Category C (AIDS indicator) condition has occurred, the person will remain in Category C.

The Impact of the 1993 Definition on Case Reporting

The CDC reported that expansion of the AIDS surveillance criteria changed both the process of AIDS surveillance and the number of reported cases. During 1993, local, state, and territorial health departments reported 103,500 AIDS cases in the United States among adults and adolescents 13 years of age and older, twice the 49,016 cases reported in 1992. Officials indicate that the increase was the one-time effect of the expansion of the AIDS definition in 1993. (See Figure 2.1.) The steep increase probably represented the reporting of persons who were diagnosed with the newly added conditions before 1993. New reported AIDS cases declined again beginning in 1996 in response to treatments that slowed the progression from HIV infection to AIDS. (See Figure 2.1.)

THE 2000 REVISED SURVEILLANCE CASE DEFINITION

On December 10, 1999, the CDC released a revised surveillance case definition, updating the definition for HIV infection implemented in 1993. (See Table 2.3.) Effective January 1, 2000, the revision integrated reporting criteria for adult and pediatric HIV infection and AIDS in a single case definition. The new definition was based on new data regarding the sensitivity and specificity of HIV diagnostic tests not available in 1993 when the AIDS definition was last revised. Newer tests detect HIV nucleic acids (DNA or RNA, viral genetic material) as opposed to previous tests that only detected anti-HIV antibodies. The newer tests allow for HIV detection in nearly all infants aged one month or older. Although reporting criteria include recommendations for diagnosing HIV infection, the primary purpose of the original and updated case definitions for HIV and AIDS is public health surveillance as opposed to the diagnosis of individual patients.

DIAGNOSIS AND SYMPTOMS OF AIDS

Only a qualified health professional can diagnose AIDS. To evaluate a patient with a positive HIV test, the health care practitioner performs a complete medical, social and family history, physical examination, and selected laboratory tests. Diagnostic laboratory testing includes: complete blood count and routine chemistry; CD4 cell count; virological assays that measure the amount of HIV-1 RNA in plasma; tuberculin skin test; along tests for syphilis, toxoplasmosis, and hepatitis B and C. Female patients are screened for cervical cancer using the cervical *Papanicolaou* ("pap") smear.

TABLE 2.2

Clinical categories of AIDS infection

Category A

Category A consists of one or more of the conditions listed below in an adolescent or adult (≥13 years) with documented HIV infection. Conditions listed in Categories B and C must not have occurred.

- Asymptomatic HIV infection
- Persistent generalized lymphadenopathy
- Acute (primary) HIV infection with accompanying illness or history of acute HIV infection

Category B

Category B consists of symptomatic conditions in an HIV-infected adolescent or adult that are not included among conditions listed in clinical Category C and that meet at least one of the following criteria: a) the conditions are attributed to HIV infection or are indicative of a defect in cell-mediated immunity; or b) the conditions are considered by physicians to have a clinical course or to require management that is complicated by HIV infection. Examples of conditions in clinical Category B include, but are not limited to:

- Bacillary angiomatosis
- Candidiasis, oropharyngeal (thrush)
- Candidiasis, vulvovaginal; persistent, frequent, or poorly responsive to therapy
- Cervical dysplasia/moderate or severe cervical carcinoma in situ
- Constitutional symptoms, such as fever (38.5 C) or diarrhea lasting >1 month
- Hairy leukoplakia, oral
- Herpes zoster (shingles), involving at least two distinct episodes or more than one dermatome
- Idiopathic thrombocytopenic purpura
- Listeriosis
- Pelvic inflammatory disease, particularly if complicated by tubo-ovarian abscess
- Peripheral neuropathy

For classification purposes, Category B conditions take precedence over those in Category A. For example, someone previously treated for oral or persistent vaginal candidiasis (and who has not developed a Category C disease) but who is now asymptomatic should be classified in clinical Category B.

Category C

Category C includes the clinical conditions listed in the AIDS surveillance case definition. For classification purposes, once a Category C condition has occurred, the person will remain in Category C.

Conditions included in the 1993 AIDS surveillance case definition

- Candidiasis of bronchi, trachea, or lungs
- Candidiasis, esophageal
- Cervical cancer, invasive*
- Coccidioidomycosis, disseminated or extrapulmonary
- Cryptococcosis, extrapulmonary
- Cryptosporidiosis, chronic intestinal (>1 month's duration)
- Cytomegalovirus disease (other than liver, spleen, or nodes)
- Cytomegalovirus retinitis (with loss of vision)
- Encephalopathy, HIV-related
- Herpes simplex: chronic ulcer(s) (>1 month's duration); or bronchitis, pneumonitis, or esophagitis
- Histoplasmosis, disseminated or extrapulmonary
- Isosporiasis, chronic intestinal (>1 month's duration)
- Kaposi's sarcoma
- Lymphoma, Burkitt's (or equivalent term)
- Lymphoma, immunoblastic (or equivalent term)
- Lymphoma, primary, of brain
- *Mycobacterium avium* complex *or M. kansasii*, disseminated or extrapulmonary
- *Mycobacterium tuberculosis*, any site (pulmonary* or extrapulmonary)
- *Mycobacterium*, other species or unidentified species, disseminated or extrapulmonary
- *Pneumocystis carinii* pneumonia
- Pneumonia, recurrent*
- Progressive multifocal leukoencephalopathy
- *Salmonella* septicemia, recurrent
- Toxoplasmosis of brain
- Wasting syndrome due to HIV

*Added in the 1993 expansion of the AIDS surveillance case definition.

SOURCE: "1993 Revised Classification System for HIV Infection and Expanded Surveillance Case Definition for AIDS Among Adolescents and Adults," *Morbidity and Mortality Weekly Report,* vol. 41, no. RR-17, December 18, 1992

HIV infection progresses through a range of stages from primary infection to a prolonged asymptomatic (symptom-free) period to advanced disease. Symptomatic patients may suffer from weight loss; malaise; nausea; fever; night sweats; swollen lymph glands; a heavy, persistent, dry cough; easy bruising or unexplained bleeding; watery diarrhea; loss of memory; balance problems; mood changes; blurring or loss of vision; and oral lesions such as thrush, a white coating of the tongue and throat. The virus is basically the same in all infected persons, but individual reactions to the virus vary greatly. Usually the opportunistic diseases, and not HIV, ultimately cause death.

FIGURE 2.1

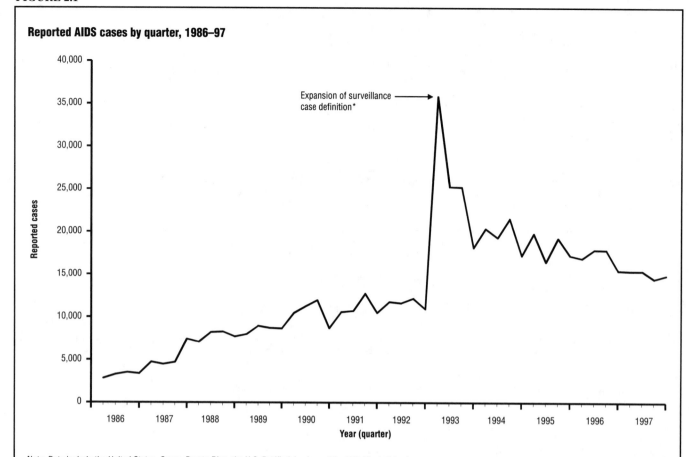

Reported AIDS cases by quarter, 1986–97

Note: Data include the United States, Guam, Puerto Rico, the U.S. Pacific Islands, and the U.S. Virgin Islands.

*The expansion of the AIDS surveillance case definition in 1993 resulted in a substantial increase in reported cases during that year. Since 1996, new treatments have slowed the progression from human immunodeficiency virus (HIV) infection to AIDS and from AIDS to death. Consequently, the number of new AIDS cases is declining, and the number of persons living with HIV infection and AIDS is increasing.

SOURCE: "Aquired Immunodeficiency Syndrome (AIDS)—reported cases by quarter, United States, 1986–1997," in "Summary of Notifiable Diseases, United States: 1997," *Morbidity and Mortality Weekly Report,* vol. 46, no. 54, November 20, 1998

Dementia

Prior to the *1987 Case Definition*, many researchers were reluctant to include dementia as a symptom indicative of AIDS. Some observers cited early studies that showed as many as 40–70 percent of persons infected with the virus developed neurological and psychological complications several years before other clinical symptoms, such as weight loss and fever, appeared. This fear had led both military and civilian authorities to bar infected persons from certain jobs involving public safety, including commercial pilots and bus drivers.

Officials of the World Health Organization (WHO), headquartered in Geneva, Switzerland, and the National Institutes of Health (NIH) in Bethesda, Maryland, jointly found these earlier estimates to be false. They reported that although neurological complications are common in the later stages of AIDS, dementia is rarely diagnosed in asymptomatic HIV-infected persons, affecting fewer than

1 percent of those infected with HIV who have not yet developed AIDS.

Research, including a U.S. Air Force study, a joint study by the CDC and the San Francisco Health Department, and the *Multicenter AIDS Cohort Study* of men who have sex with men (MSM) in Baltimore, Chicago, Los Angeles, and Pittsburgh (sponsored by the National Institute of Allergy and Infectious Diseases and the National Cancer Institute), found far lower rates of dementia than those reported in earlier studies. One explanation for the higher, earlier figures may have been that the research data came from centers to which AIDS patients with dementia had been referred for treatment. Today HIV-associated dementia (also called AIDS dementia complex) is recognized as declining cognitive function that generally occurs in the late stages of HIV infection. Sometimes symptoms of dementia such as forgetfulness and difficulty concentrating are not easily distinguished from depression and fatigue.

TABLE 2.3

Revised Surveillance Case Definition for HIV Infection[1]

This revised definition of HIV infection, which applies to any HIV (e.g., HIV-1 or HIV-2), is intended for public health surveillance only. It incorporates the reporting criteria for HIV infection and AIDS into a single case definition. The revised criteria for HIV infection update the definition of HIV infection implemented in 1993; the revised HIV criteria apply to AIDS-defining conditions for adults and children, which require laboratory evidence of HIV. This definition is **not** presented as a guide to clinical diagnosis or for other uses.

I. **In adults, adolescents, or children aged ≥18 months[2], a reportable case of HIV infection must meet at least one of the following criteria:**

   Laboratory Criteria:
   Positive result on a screening test for HIV antibody (e.g., repeatedly reactive enzyme immunoassay), followed by a positive result on a confirmatory (sensitive and more specific) test for HIV antibody (e.g., Western blot or immunofluorescence antibody test)
   or
   Positive result or report of a detectable quantity on any of the following HIV virologic (nonantibody) tests:
   - HIV nucleic acid (DNA or RNA) detection (e.g., DNA polymerase chain reaction [PCR] or plasma HIV-1 RNA)[3]
   - HIV p24 antigen test, including neutralization assay
   - HIV isolation (viral culture)

   OR
   Clinical or Other Criteria (if the above laboratory criteria are not met)
   Diagnosis of HIV infection, based on the laboratory criteria above, that is documented in a medical record by a physician
   or
   Conditions that meet criteria included in the case definition for AIDS

II. **In a child aged <18 months, a reportable case of HIV infection must meet at least one of the following criteria:**
   Laboratory Criteria
   Definitive
   Positive results on two separate specimens (excluding cord blood) using one or more of the following HIV virologic (nonantibody) tests:
   - HIV nucleic acid (DNA or RNA) detection
   - HIV p24 antigen test, including neutralization assay, in a child ≥1 month of age
   - HIV isolation (viral culture)

   or

   Presumptive
   A child who does not meet the criteria for definitive HIV infection but who has:
   Positive results on only one specimen (excluding cord blood) using the above HIV virologic tests and no subsequent negative HIV virologic or negative HIV antibody tests

   OR
   Clinical or Other Criteria (if the above definitive or presumptive laboratory criteria are not met)
   Diagnosis of HIV infection, based on the laboratory criteria above, that is documented in a medical record by a physician
   or
   Conditions that meet criteria included in the 1987 pediatric surveillance case definition for AIDS

From HIV to AIDS

By 2001 the average amount of time from initial HIV infection to the development of AIDS was 11 years, although there are cases in which patients have been HIV-positive for up to 20 years before developing AIDS. At one time death normally followed within two years of being diagnosed with AIDS. Medical developments during the 1980s and 1990s, however, have significantly increased the life expectancy of AIDS patients.

THE EARLY STAGE. The timing and details of the HIV infection vary widely with individuals, but the disease follows a basic pattern. In the beginning of the early stage, the T4 cell count is normal, at around 1,000 per cubic millimeter. The virus enters the bloodstream, although it cannot be detected by antibody testing for up to six weeks and in some unusual cases may take a year or more to appear. Many people, even after testing positive for the virus, remain asymptomatic (showing no symptoms) for a long time, although they may develop a disorder similar to infectious mononucleosis with fatigue, fever, swollen glands, and possibly a rash. Often these symptoms disappear within a few weeks. Throughout this time, the virus is quietly multiplying, destroying healthy cells. Most people continue to feel fine, though some may have chronically swollen lymph nodes. This stage usually lasts about five years.

THE MIDDLE STAGE. By the middle stage, the CD4+ T cell count is reduced by half to around 500, though many people may still be asymptomatic. As the infection advances, skin tests will likely show that cell-mediated immunity, a form of immunological defense, is disintegrating. This stage can also last up to five years.

AZT (originally azidothymidine; now called zidovudine), a failed cancer drug, was introduced in the mid-1980s, garnering mass publicity because it helped keep HIV from attaching itself to host cells and delayed the onset of symptoms, promising to extend this middle stage. The benefits of this antiretroviral drug, however, proved to be temporary. HIV mutates so rapidly that it eludes AZT. The drug is still used today in conjunction with other medicines, and some studies suggest that people who receive AZT may develop AIDS later than those who do not take AZT. Newer and possibly better drugs have since been developed, the most promising of which are protease inhibitors (which received FDA approval in December 1995) and Structured Treatment Interruptions (STIs), initially proposed in the late 1990s.

TABLE 2.3

Revised Surveillance Case Definition for HIV Infection[1] [CONTINUED]

III. **A child aged <18 months born to an HIV-infected mother will be categorized for surveillance purposes as "not infected with HIV" if the child does not meet the criteria for HIV infection but meets the following criteria:**
Laboratory Criteria
Definitive
    At least two negative HIV antibody tests from separate specimens obtained at ≥6 months of age
or

    At least two negative HIV virologic tests[4] from separate specimens, both of which were performed at ≥1 month of age and one of which was performed at ≥4 months of age

AND

No other laboratory or clinical evidence of HIV infection (i.e., has not had any positive virologic tests, if performed, and has not had an AIDS-defining condition)
or

Presumptive
A child who does not meet the above criteria for definitive "not infected" status but who has:
    One negative EIA HIV antibody test performed at ≥6 months of age and NO positive HIV virologic tests, if performed
or

    One negative HIV virologic test[4] performed at ≥4 months of age and NO positive HIV virologic tests, if performed
or

    One positive HIV virologic test with at least two subsequent negative virologic tests[4], at least one of which is at ≥4 months of age; or negative HIV antibody test results, at least one of which is at ≥6 months of age

AND

No other laboratory or clinical evidence of HIV infection (i.e., has not had any positive virologic tests, if performed, and has not had an AIDS-defining condition).
OR
Clinical or Other Criteria (if the above definitive or presumptive laboratory criteria are not met)
    Determined by a physician to be "not infected", and a physician has noted the results of the preceding HIV diagnostic tests in the medical record
AND

NO other laboratory or clinical evidence of HIV infection (i.e., has not had any positive virologic tests, if performed, and has not had an AIDS-defining condition)

IV. **A child aged <18 months born to an HIV-infected mother will be categorized as having perinatal exposure to HIV infection if the child does not meet the criteria for HIV infection (II) or the criteria for "not infected with HIV" (III).**

[1] Draft revised surveillance criteria for HIV infection were approved and recommended by the membership of the Council of State and Territorial Epidemiologists (CSTE) at the 1998 annual meeting. Draft versions of these criteria were previously reviewed by state HIV/AIDS surveillance staffs, CDC, CSTE, and laboratory experts. In addition, the pediatric criteria were reviewed by an expert panel of consultants. [External Pediatric Consultants: C. Hanson, M. Kaiser, S. Paul, G. Scott, and P. Thomas. CDC staff: J. Bertolli, K. Dominguez, M. Kalish, M.L. Lindegren, M. Rogers, C. Schable, R.J. Simonds, and J. Ward]
[2] Children aged ≥18 months but <13 years are categorized as "not infected with HIV" if they meet the criteria in **III**.
[3] In adults, adolescents, and children infected by other than perinatal exposure, plasma viral RNA nucleic acid tests should **NOT** be used in lieu of licensed HIV screening tests (e.g., repeatedly reactive enzyme immunoassay). In addition, a negative (i.e., undetectable) plasma HIV-1 RNA test result does not rule out the diagnosis of HIV infection.
[4] HIV nucleic acid (DNA or RNA) detection tests are the virologic methods of choice to exclude infection in children aged <18 months. Although HIV culture can be used for this purpose, it is more complex and expensive to perform and is less well standardized than nucleic acid detection tests. The use of p24 antigen testing to exclude infection in children aged <18 months is not recommended because of its lack of sensitivity.

SOURCE: "Revised Surveillance Case Definition for HIV Infection," in *CDC Guidelines for National Human Immunodeficiency Virus Case Surveillance Including Monitoring for HIV and AIDS,* MMWR vol. 48, no. RR-13, December 10, 1999

THE LATE STAGE. The third and final stage is reached when the CD4+ T cell count drops to 200 or below. Though many patients are still asymptomatic at this point, the risk of bacteria, viruses, fungi, parasites, and cancer taking advantage of their weakened immune systems increases dramatically. In order to prevent PCP, one of the most common opportunistic infections, patients are usually treated with antibiotics during this stage. Early in this stage, patients may experience weight loss, diarrhea, lethargy, and fevers. Skin and mucous membrane infections increase. Oral fungal infections such as thrush, in which white spots and ulcers appear on the tongue and mouth, and chronic herpes simplex are common.

The immune system begins to collapse rapidly, allowing opportunistic infections to move deeper into the body. It is not uncommon for a parasitic infection called toxoplasmosis to attack the brain, while the cryptococcosis fungus attacks the nervous system, liver, bones, and skin. Cytomegalovirus (CMV) can cause pneumonia, encephalitis, and retinitis, an inflammation of the retina that can cause blindness. The list of possible infections, consequences, and complications of compromised immune function is virtually endless. The late stage lasts an average of two years.

TRANSMISSION

When AIDS was first discovered, it was often compared to the Black Death of the fourteenth century. That disease, however, was readily transmitted via food, water, and air. HIV/AIDS is not nearly as contagious as the Black Death or many other infectious diseases and is almost entirely preventable.

More than 20 years of research and observation have definitively concluded that the HIV infection can only be transmitted:

- By oral, anal, or vaginal sex with an infected person (worldwide, heterosexual sex is the most common mode of transmission).

- By sharing drug needles or syringes with an infected person.

- From an infected mother to her baby perinatally (at the time of birth) and possibly though breast milk.

- By receiving a transplanted organ or bodily fluids, such as blood transfusions or blood products, from an infected person.

High concentrations of HIV have been found in blood, semen, and cerebrospinal fluid. Concentrations 1,000 times less have been found in saliva, tears, vaginal secretions, breast milk, and feces. There have been no reports, however, of HIV transmission from saliva, tears, or human bites. In fact, in 1995 the National Institute of Dental Research in Bethesda, Maryland, reported that a small protein found in human saliva actually blocks the virus from entering the system.

Casual Contact

While HIV is an infectious, contagious disease, it is not spread in the same manner as a common cold or chicken pox. It is not spread by sneezing or coughing, as are airborne illnesses. HIV is not spread by sharing a bathroom or swimming pool or by hugging or shaking hands. Studies of family members who lived with and cared for AIDS patients have not found definitive evidence that anyone has become infected through casual contact. Still, myths abound. To combat misinformation the U.S. Surgeon General's office and public health education initiatives continue to stress that HIV is *not* spread by:

- Bites from mosquitoes or other insects.

- Bites from animals.

- Food handled, prepared, or served by HIV-infected persons.

- Forks, spoons, knives, or drinking glasses used by HIV-infected persons.

- Chairs previously occupied by persons with HIV.

- Casual contact such as touching, hugging, or kissing a person who is HIV-positive. (Open-mouth kissing with a person who is HIV-positive is not recommended because of potential exposure to blood.)

Donating Blood

Health officials agree that donating blood poses no danger of HIV infection for the donors. The needles used to draw blood from donors are new and are thrown away after one use. Contact with HIV from donating blood is therefore impossible.

SAFETY OF BLOOD AND TRANSPLANT PROCEDURES

According to the CDC, more than 400 establishments either bank or commercially process one or more human tissues, organs, or fluids. Approximately 100 eye banks, 125 bone banks, 100 semen banks, 99 bone marrow transplant centers, and 7 human milk banks operate in the United States, although the number of hospitals that store bone and the number of physicians' offices that store semen are undetermined.

To safeguard the nation's transplant recipients, the CDC has suggested that all donors of blood products, tissue, and organs be screened and tested. The recommendations include screening for behaviors—risk factors—associated with acquisition of HIV infection, a physical examination for signs and symptoms related to HIV infection, and laboratory screening for antibodies to HIV. It is important to remember that the CDC does not regulate medical protocol; its main function is to offer health care guidelines and information to the nation and its health care providers.

The U.S. Blood Supply

Before HIV-antibody testing began in 1985, it is estimated that 70 percent of hemophiliacs (people with inherited bleeding disorders) who received blood products were given tainted blood-clotting factor (a concentrate of blood used to stem bleeding) and infected with HIV. Approximately 10,000 of these patients developed AIDS and, according to the National Hemophilia Foundation, most have died.

Widespread use of two blood-screening tests, both of which are also used on plasma and other blood products, has resulted in the consensus that the U.S. blood and plasma supply is safer than it has ever been. Since 1992 the U.S. Public Health Service, an arm of the U.S. Department of Health and Human Services, has required that all blood and plasma donations be screened for the rare HIV-2 antibody, as well as the more common HIV-1 antibody.

In 2001 the FDA approved the first nucleic acid test (NAT) system to screen plasma donors for HIV. Rather than relying on the identification of antigens or antibodies, the new test provides extremely sensitive detection of RNA from HIV-1. Even with the new test there is still some risk, however, due to the "window period" during which a person who has acquired the HIV-1 infection may still test negative. For HIV-1, the window period ranges from 16 days for antigen testing to 22 days for antibody tests; NAT systems reduce the window period to 12 days. Of the 12 million units of blood donated annually, the CDC estimates that between 32 and 49 units are potentially infectious. While the nation's blood supply is considered to be safe, blood banks across the country encourage individuals concerned about tainted blood to bank their own blood for possible future use.

Foreign Blood Supply

HIV infection from contaminated blood is much more common in other countries. In July 1998 a French court ruled that a former Prime Minister and two former cabinet members would be tried on charges that they allowed

HIV-contaminated blood to be used for transfusions during 1984 and 1985. Relatives of the patients argued that the French government had refused American technology that would have detected antibodies in the tainted blood in favor of a French procedure in development. Estimates vary, but as many as 4,000 persons acquired HIV as a result of this action. An estimated 1,250 hemophiliacs were infected and at least 400 of them, including many children, have since died of AIDS. The former French officials, Prime Minister Fabius, former Social Affairs Minister Georgina Dufoix, and former Health Minister Edmond Herve, faced charges of involuntary homicide and went to trial in 1999. Herve was convicted without a penalty and Dufoix and Fabius were acquitted.

In 1995 the WHO reported that 3,000 children in Romania—home to thousands of abandoned babies left in squalid institutions after the fall of Romanian dictator Nicolae Ceausescu—were infected by contaminated blood and syringes in the late 1980s. WHO estimates that 1,000 of those children have died. In 1998 Romania had more than half of the juvenile AIDS cases in Europe; more than 90 percent of the country's AIDS cases are among children. The Romanian Health Ministry faced litigation for causing the spread of HIV.

In 1995 the owner of a German drug laboratory was charged with nearly 6,000 counts of murder or attempted murder for selling HIV-tainted blood products to German hospitals in 1987. Not all of the 6,000 batches distributed had been tested for HIV. Testing has been mandatory in Germany since 1986.

Organ and Tissue Transplants

In several instances HIV has been transmitted through organ (kidney, liver, heart, lung, and pancreas) and other tissue transplants. The risk of such transmission is low simply because there are far fewer transplant cases than blood transfusions.

In 1994 the Food and Drug Administration (FDA) began regulating the sale of bone, skin, corneas, cartilage, tendons, and similar non-blood-vessel-bearing tissues used for transplants. The FDA requires that all procurement agencies conduct behavioral screening and infectious-disease (HIV-1, HIV-2, hepatitis B virus, and hepatitis C virus) testing of donors.

TESTING PEOPLE FOR HIV

A person infected with HIV produces antibodies (proteins intended to neutralize the virus) to that virus. While the antibodies are not enough to successfully fight HIV, they do indicate the presence of the virus. HIV testing is done for HIV antibodies rather than for the virus itself because it is too difficult to isolate the virus from the blood. Testing serves two purposes: first, it determines if

there is any viral infection in blood, tissue, or organ donors; second, donor testing protects transfusion and transplant recipients from the virus.

The test cannot detect all HIV-positive blood. Unfortunately, it can take between 4 and 12 weeks following HIV infection for antibodies to appear. This interval between acquisition of the virus and the appearance of antibodies is sometimes referred to as the "window period." In some reported cases, HIV antibodies have taken up to one year to appear. Consequently it is possible that some HIV-infected donors may not be diagnosed and their blood may enter the nation's blood supply. In addition to the diagnostic laboratory tests, blood banks routinely question potential donors about high-risk behaviors. Any donor whose behavior might indicate an increased risk of HIV infection (for example, intravenous drug use or male-to-male sex) is automatically excluded from donating blood.

Diagnostic Tools

Two tests commonly used to detect HIV antibodies are believed to be about 99 percent reliable. The enzyme-linked immunosorbent assay (ELISA), a test designed for screening rather than diagnosing, was introduced in 1985. The assay contains HIV antigens and determines if a patient's blood contains antibodies to these antigens. A sample of blood is added to proteins from the AIDS virus. If antibodies are present, they attach themselves to the viral proteins, and through chemical reactions, the color of the mixture changes. This test is simple to conduct and inexpensive.

The Western blot, introduced in 1987, is a confirmatory test commonly used to verify the results of the less-specific assays. The Western blot technique places various HIV proteins on a membrane strip. The blood sample is then applied to the membrane. If HIV antibodies are present in the blood sample, they will bind to the HIV proteins. Chemicals that produce bands of color wherever antibodies have adhered to viral proteins are then added. The Western blot provides a positive, negative, or intermediate result. The presence of three or more of the color bands confirms infection with the HIV. (See Figure 2.2.) If fewer—one or two— bands appear, the test is considered intermediate and retesting is performed six months later. If no color bands appear, the test is considered negative with no HIV present, though many who test negative also repeat the test six months later.

Urine Tests

In June 1998 the FDA approved a new, urine-based diagnostic kit for HIV that does not require confirmation by blood test. Urine tests are easier to use and cost less than blood tests for health care providers. According to the NIH, there is no evidence that HIV is spread through urine. Therefore, the chances of accidental infection through needle sticks or handling of samples are lessened.

The urine test and its urine-based confirmation test, like most blood tests, recognize the existence of antibodies, not the actual virus.

Calypte Biomedical Corporation, a producer of the urine test, markets the test to life insurance companies, clinical laboratories, public health agencies, the military, immigration, and the criminal justice system. In June 2000 Calypte announced its partnership with the Chinese National Center for AIDS Prevention and Control (NCAIDS) to distribute the first HIV-1 antibody urine test in the People's Republic of China. NCAIDS estimates that the total number of HIV infections in China could rise as high as 10 million before 2010 if proper counter-measures are not taken. The Chinese plan to use the Calypte product as the exclusive non-invasive method of testing for HIV.

Home Testing

In 1997 a recently approved home HIV test was analyzed in a multi-site test study involving 1,255 people. Test participants registered anonymously by telephone with a testing laboratory. The subjects simply stuck a finger to draw blood and mailed the dried blood sample on filter paper to the laboratory. There a phlebotomist (a health worker who draws blood by syringe or needle) matched the results with blood that had been drawn earlier from the patient's vein in the traditional manner. Results of the test were obtained by calling a toll-free telephone number. Negative results were given by recorded message. For positive results, a trained counselor offered callers follow-up information and counseling. Of the 1,255 people who participated, 1,104 participants called in to check their test results. For those participants the home test matched the phlebotomy results exactly.

Although there is no new technology involved in home testing, it offers the advantages of privacy and ease of use. Critics of home testing point out that it is expensive; a kit costs $40 to $60 and may be prohibitively expensive for poorer populations—for whom such a test is most needed. Critics also question the impersonal practice of relaying HIV-positive results and follow-up counseling by telephone.

As of 2001 the FDA had approved only the Home Access Express HIV Test System, produced by the Home Access Health Corporation. The FDA warned that non-approved home HIV tests could produce inaccurate results. When Home Access testing kits were placed on store shelves (rather than behind pharmacy counters) in 1998, two retail drugstore chains reported sales increases for the tests ranging from 360 to 570 percent.

Quick Response Tests

During the mid-to-late 1990s, the CDC recommended the development of a new HIV test that would give results

FIGURE 2.2

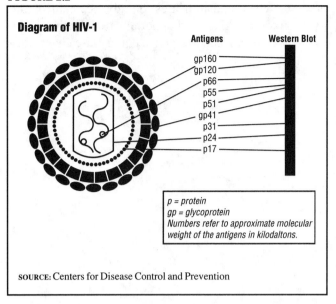

Diagram of HIV-1

Antigens — Western Blot

gp160, gp120, p66, p55, p51, gp41, p31, p24, p17

p = protein
gp = glycoprotein
Numbers refer to approximate molecular weight of the antigens in kilodaltons.

SOURCE: Centers for Disease Control and Prevention

instantly rather than taking a week. The CDC hoped that this would encourage people to learn the results of their tests. Currently nearly 700,000 people each year do not follow up to learn their test results. The proposed test would make it possible for people to receive immediate education and treatment.

The FDA has approved one rapid test to be used in clinics in the United States. It is manufactured by Murex Diagnostics, Inc., of Norcross, Georgia, and determines in about 10 minutes whether the virus is present. The test is as accurate as the standard test. This new test, like the old tests, looks for antibodies in the blood. However, tests that traditionally take one week to give results also look for protein bands, the absolute indicator of HIV.

The CDC stresses the importance of obtaining results quickly. They contend that people are not only more likely to take a test that gives results instantly but also will benefit from the opportunity to learn they are infected before their immune systems have been seriously damaged. Further, rapid results may lead to earlier, more effective treatment and might reduce transmission of the virus.

Rapid HIV tests are used more frequently in other countries. In Third World countries, quick response tests are used to screen blood before transfusions, to screen pregnant women so medical interventions can be given to prevent mother-to-child transmission of the virus, and in rural clinics.

Test Tracks HIV/AIDS Progression

In June 1996 the FDA approved a test to help determine how fast an HIV infection is progressing to full-blown AIDS. Developed by Roche Diagnostic Systems, Inc., the Amplicor HIV-1 monitor test is not intended to screen for HIV or to confirm an HIV diagnosis. Instead the test detects the amount of HIV in the blood by measuring HIV genetic material, or viral load. An increased viral load indicates the advancement of the infection toward AIDS and opportunistic infections. The test is based on a technique called polymerase chain reaction (PCR), developed in 1984, which allows rapid production of millions of copies of genetic material from microbes within minutes to hours. This test is the first PCR-based test to be approved.

CHAPTER 3

PATTERNS AND TRENDS IN HIV/AIDS SURVEILLANCE

DETERMINING THE NUMBER OF PERSONS INFECTED WITH HIV

The Centers for Disease Control and Prevention (CDC) is an organization that estimates the number of persons in the United States who are infected with HIV, the virus that causes AIDS. These figures are sometimes criticized as being either too high or too low. The CDC acknowledges that many of its findings are no more than estimates. CDC data through December 2000 from the 33 states with confidential HIV reporting found that 127,058 persons are living with HIV which has not yet progressed to AIDS. (See Table 3.1.) Of these, 1,608 are children less than 13 years old and 125,450 are adults and adolescents. The December 2000 data also indicated that among all the U.S. states and territories (Guam, Pacific Islands, Puerto Rico, and Virgin Islands), a total of 322,865 people are living with AIDS (including 2,703 children less than 13 years old and 320,161 adults and adolescents).

Estimates of HIV infection directly affect public health, medical resource allocation, political, and economic decisions. Accurate estimates, however, are difficult to obtain because laws prevent testing for HIV without consent and permission. Further, many people are understandably reluctant to participate in household surveys because of confidentiality concerns and fear of losing or failing to get insurance coverage.

Health officials contend that knowing the prevalence of HIV infections (prevalence is a measure of all cases of illness existing at a given point in time) is not as crucial as knowing whether the number of HIV infections is rising or falling. The rate at which people develop HIV/AIDS during a specified period of time is known as the incidence rate. Since there are no national studies to collect this data (not all states require reporting of new HIV cases), estimates are based on reports from states that mandate confidential reporting of HIV cases, along with other small studies and surveys. Officials with the CDC explain that a major problem has been lack of knowledge about how many people have become infected over the past five years. This would help to determine how the incidence of HIV in 2000 compares to previous years. Comparison of incidence rates is important because they are a direct measure of the rate at which individuals become ill and provide data to help estimate the risk or probability of illness.

AIDS CASE NUMBERS

The first cases in the United States of what is now known as AIDS were reported in June 1981 when five young homosexual males in Los Angeles were diagnosed with *Pneumocystis carinii* pneumonia (PCP) and other opportunistic infections (OIs). By August 1989 approximately 100,000 cases of AIDS had been reported to the CDC. By December 1997 that number had risen to 641,086; of these, 390,692 people had died. As of December 2000 the total of all reported cases was 765,559, and 448,060 of these people had died. (See Table 3.2.)

During the mid-1990s, the number of AIDS cases rose dramatically. This surge was a result of the expanded 1993 AIDS surveillance definition which added diseases and conditions that had not been part of the prior definition of AIDS. The new definition, as opposed to the natural course of the epidemic, was responsible for the sharp increase in the number of cases reported during the mid-1990s. By the late 1990s, the number of cases leveled off and began to decline, probably as a result of increasing use of effective antiretroviral drugs that delay the progression of AIDS. The number of new cases (42,156) reported between 1999 and December 2000 was lower than the 47,083 reported in the period between 1998 and 1999.

THE NATURE OF THE EPIDEMIC

The changes in the distribution of those infected with HIV illustrate the increasing diversity of persons affected

TABLE 3.1

Persons reported to be living with HIV infection and with AIDS, by area and age group,[1] December 2000[2]

Area of residence (Date HIV reporting initiated)	Living with HIV infection[3]			Living with AIDS[4]			Cumulative totals		
	Adults/ adolescents	Children <13 years old	Total	Adults/ adolescents	Children <13 years old	Total	Adults/ adolescents	Children <13 years old	Total
Alabama (Jan. 1988)	5,014	32	5,046	3,142	17	3,159	8,156	49	8,205
Alaska (Feb. 1999)	29	—	29	229	1	230	258	1	259
Arizona (Jan. 1987)	4,296	28	4,324	3,217	9	3,226	7,513	37	7,550
Arkansas (July 1989)	2,001	15	2,016	1,612	20	1,632	3,613	35	3,648
California	—	—	—	43,606	155	43,761	43,606	155	43,761
Colorado (Nov. 1985)	5,265	18	5,283	2,878	1	2,879	8,143	19	8,162
Connecticut (July 1992)[5]	—	74	74	5,788	58	5,846	5,788	132	5,920
Delaware	—	—	—	1,193	13	1,206	1,193	13	1,206
District of Columbia	—	—	—	6,389	84	6,473	6,389	84	6,473
Florida (July 1997)	18,774	165	18,939	35,195	475	35,670	53,969	640	54,609
Georgia	—	—	—	10,206	84	10,290	10,206	84	10,290
Hawaii	—	—	—	982	5	987	982	5	987
Idaho (June 1986)	321	3	324	223	—	223	544	3	547
Illinois	—	—	—	9,761	107	9,868	9,761	107	9,868
Indiana (July 1988)	3,252	27	3,279	2,693	13	2,706	5,945	40	5,985
Iowa (July 1998)	354	5	359	573	5	578	927	10	937
Kansas (July 1999)	930	10	940	980	3	983	1,910	13	1,923
Kentucky	—	—	—	1,619	14	1,633	1,619	14	1,633
Louisiana (Feb. 1993)	6,975	88	7,063	5,448	49	5,497	12,423	137	12,560
Maine	—	—	—	441	5	446	441	5	446
Maryland	—	—	—	9,933	129	10,062	9,933	129	10,062
Massachusetts	—	—	—	6,770	58	6,828	6,770	58	6,828
Michigan (April 1992)	4,611	73	4,684	4,618	23	4,641	9,229	96	9,325
Minnesota (Oct. 1985)	2,552	24	2,576	1,632	9	1,641	4,184	33	4,217
Mississippi (Aug. 1988)	4,104	38	4,142	2,102	23	2,125	6,206	61	6,267
Missouri (Oct. 1987)	4,159	35	4,194	4,263	16	4,279	8,422	51	8,473
Montana	—	—	—	165	—	165	165	—	165
Nebraska (Sept. 1995)	474	5	479	482	4	486	956	9	965
Nevada (Feb. 1992)	2,591	21	2,612	2,084	10	2,094	4,675	31	4,706
New Hampshire	—	—	—	478	4	482	478	4	482
New Jersey (Jan. 1992)	12,367	314	12,681	14,910	185	15,095	27,277	499	27,776
New Mexico (Jan. 1998)	630	—	630	956	6	962	1,586	6	1,592
New York	—	—	—	54,290	503	54,794	54,290	503	54,794
North Carolina (Feb. 1990)	9,133	93	9,226	4,511	37	4,548	13,644	130	13,774
North Dakota (Jan. 1988)	63	1	64	44	1	45	107	2	109
Ohio (June 1990)	5,409	54	5,463	4,487	36	4,523	9,896	90	9,986
Oklahoma (June 1988)	2,239	11	2,250	1,574	6	1,580	3,813	17	3,830
Oregon (Sept. 1988)[5]	—	13	13	2,022	5	2,027	2,022	18	2,040
Pennsylvania	—	—	—	11,487	152	11,639	11,487	152	11,639
Rhode Island	—	—	—	893	6	899	893	6	899
South Carolina (Feb. 1986)	6,367	82	6,449	4,696	26	4,722	11,063	108	11,171
South Dakota (Jan. 1988)	188	1	189	69	1	70	257	2	259
Tennessee (Jan. 1992)	5,624	54	5,678	4,701	17	4,718	10,325	71	10,396
Texas (Jan. 1999)[5]	6,640	236	6,876	23,869	125	23,994	30,509	361	30,870
Utah (April 1989)	711	6	717	993	3	996	1,704	9	1,713
Vermont	—	—	—	194	2	196	194	2	196
Virginia (July 1989)	7,611	61	7,672	5,774	69	5,843	13,385	130	13,515
Washington	—	—	—	4,083	11	4,094	4,083	11	4,094
West Virginia (Jan. 1989)	555	4	559	465	4	469	1,020	8	1,028
Wisconsin (Nov. 1985)	2,145	17	2,162	1,549	11	1,560	3,694	28	3,722
Wyoming (June 1989)	66	—	66	75	1	76	141	1	142
Subtotal	**125,450**	**1,608**	**127,058**	**310,344**	**2,601**	**312,946**	**435,794**	**4,210**	**440,004**
U.S. dependencies, possessions, and associated nations									
Guam (March 2000)	41	1	42	24	—	24	65	1	66
Pacific Islands, U.S.	—	—	—	2	—	2	2	—	2
Puerto Rico	—	—	—	9,204	89	9,293	9,204	89	9,293
Virgin Isl, U.S.(Dec.1998)	184	2	186	212	7	219	396	9	405
Total	125,675	1,611	127,286	320,161	2,703	322,865	445,836	4,314	450,151

[1]Age group based on person's age as of December 31, 2000.
[2]Persons reported with vital status "alive" as of the last update. Excludes persons whose vital status is unknown.
[3]Includes only persons reported with HIV infection who have not developed AIDS. Includes only persons reported from areas with confidential HIV reporting. Excludes 2,160 adults/ adolescents and 51 children reported from areas with confidential HIV infection reporting whose area of residence is unknown or are residents of other areas.
[4]Includes 375 adults/adolescents and 6 children whose area of residence is unknown, and one person missing age.
[5]Connecticut has confidential HIV infection reporting for pediatric cases only; Oregon has confidential HIV infection reporting for children less than 6 years old. Texas reported only pediatric HIV infection cases from February 1994 until January 1999.

SOURCE: "Table 1. Persons reported to be living with HIV infection and with AIDS, by area and age group, reported through December 2000," in *HIV/AIDS Surveillance Report,* vol. 12, no. 2, Centers for Disease Control and Prevention, Atlanta, GA, 2000

TABLE 3.2

Deaths in persons with AIDS, by various characteristics, occurring in 1998 and 1999; and cumulative totals reported through December 2000[1]

Race/ethnicity and age at death[2]	Males			Females			Both sexes[3]		
	1998	1999	Cumulative total	1998	1999	Cumulative total	1998	1999	Cumulative total
White, not Hispanic									
Under 15	6	7	568	6	4	422	12	11	990
15-24	33	19	2,541	11	12	480	44	31	3,021
25-34	869	598	54,902	156	132	4,692	1,025	730	59,594
35-44	2,202	1,710	81,121	288	281	5,213	2,490	1,991	86,335
45-54	1,328	1,169	37,252	127	141	2,052	1,455	1,310	39,304
55 or older	561	475	15,732	62	51	1,751	623	526	17,483
All ages	4,999	3,978	192,276	650	621	14,632	5,649	4,599	206,909
Black, not Hispanic									
Under 15	30	37	1,444	48	28	1,424	78	65	2,868
15-24	70	51	2,459	87	76	1,447	157	127	3,906
25-34	1,073	859	33,731	648	548	11,968	1,721	1,407	45,699
35-44	2,324	2,156	50,579	1,014	993	15,121	3,338	3,149	65,700
45-54	1,605	1,561	22,923	510	507	5,465	2,115	2,068	28,388
55 or older	699	690	9,768	214	215	2,406	913	905	12,174
All ages	5,801	5,354	121,030	2,521	2,367	37,862	8,322	7,721	158,892
Hispanic									
Under 15	10	10	632	9	14	583	19	24	1,215
15-24	31	18	1,342	12	17	486	43	35	1,828
25-34	509	416	20,387	179	148	4,580	688	564	24,967
35-44	1,059	900	26,518	276	277	5,013	1,335	1,177	31,531
45-54	576	502	10,859	127	154	1,846	703	656	12,705
55 or older	276	261	4,514	68	46	874	344	307	5,388
All ages	2,461	2,107	64,305	671	656	13,393	3,132	2,763	77,698
Asian/Pacific Islander									
Under 15	—	—	19	—	1	16	—	1	35
15-24	1	2	37	—	1	6	1	3	43
25-34	28	12	720	6	5	82	34	17	802
35-44	39	42	1,141	8	1	104	47	43	1,245
45-54	18	21	551	3	7	67	21	28	618
55 or older	11	7	254	4	2	54	15	9	308
All ages	97	84	2,724	21	17	331	118	101	3,055
American Indian/Alaska Native									
Under 15	—	—	12	—	—	8	—	—	20
15-24	—	—	26	—	—	3	—	—	29
25-34	20	12	388	6	3	74	26	15	462
35-44	21	17	405	8	7	73	29	24	478
45-54	9	12	137	1	1	29	10	13	166
55 or older	6	2	46	—	3	13	6	5	59
All ages	56	43	1,017	15	14	200	71	57	1,217
All racial/ethnic groups									
Under 15	46	54	2,677	63	47	2,454	109	101	5,131
15-24	135	90	6,410	110	106	2,424	245	196	8,834
25-34	2,501	1,899	110,187	995	836	21,402	3,496	2,735	131,589
35-44	5,651	4,831	159,883	1,595	1,561	25,537	7,246	6,392	185,421
45-54	3,539	3,268	71,770	768	810	9,464	4,307	4,078	81,234
55 or older	1,553	1,435	30,338	348	317	5,101	1,901	1,752	35,439
All ages	13,425	11,577	381,611	3,879	3,677	66,448	17,304	15,254	448,060

[1]Data tabulations for 1998 and 1999 are based on date of death occurrence. Data for deaths occurring in 2000 are incomplete and not tabulated separately, but are included in the cumulative totals. Tabulations for 1998 and 1999 may increase as additional deaths are reported to CDC.
[2]Data tabulated under "all ages" include 412 persons whose age at death is unknown. Data tabulated under "all racial/ethnic groups" include 289 persons whose race/ethnicity is unknown.
[3]Includes 1 person whose sex is unknown.

SOURCE: "Table 20. Deaths in persons with AIDS, by race/ethnicity, age at death, and sex, occurring in 1998 and 1999; and cumulative totals reported through December 2000, United States," in *HIV/AIDS Surveillance Report*, vol. 12, no. 2, Centers for Disease Control and Prevention, Atlanta, GA, 2000

by the HIV epidemic in the more than 20 years since AIDS was first diagnosed. In 1981, all of the 189 AIDS cases reported in the United States were males. Three-fourths of these were men who have sex with men (MSM) living in New York and California. In 1990, of the more than 43,000 AIDS cases reported by all states, only one-third were from New York and California, 11 percent were women, and approximately 800 were children. In 1999 the proportions of reported cases increased among women, African Americans, Hispanics, and persons exposed through heterosexual contact. On the other hand, the percentage of reported cases among whites and MSM declined somewhat.

Regional Differences

Although AIDS cases have been reported in all 50 states, the District of Columbia, and four U.S. territories, the distribution of cases is far from even. Between 1999 and 2000 annual incidence rates varied from 0.5 cases per 100,000 persons in North Dakota to 153 cases per 100,000 persons in the District of Columbia. Most recently reported cases were concentrated on the East Coast (particularly New York and Florida), in California, and in Texas. (See Table 3.3.) Figure 3.1 shows the distribution of male and female adult/adolescent HIV infection and AIDS cases reported by state in 2000.

RATES IN MAJOR METROPOLITAN AREAS. The majority of AIDS cases are concentrated in larger metropolitan regions (including the city as well as surrounding suburban areas). Metropolitan areas with populations of 500,000 or more accounted for more than 80 percent of all reported cases between 1999 and 2000 and 84 percent of cumulative (including those who have died and those who survive) totals since 1981. AIDS incidence rates per 100,000 were highest on the coasts, such as in New York City (56.6), Fort Lauderdale (53) Miami (58), West Palm Beach (48.2), and San Francisco (44.2). On the other hand, metropolitan areas in the Midwest—Akron, Ohio (4.3), Grand Rapids, Michigan (3.3), and Youngstown, Ohio (3.0)—experienced the lowest rates. Youngstown and Scranton, Pennsylvania had the lowest overall rate (3.0) of all metropolitan areas. (See Table 3.4.)

There are several reasons for the higher rates in the above-mentioned urban areas. First, metropolitan areas are more cosmopolitan and, by definition, more tolerant of alternative lifestyles such as those of MSM, a group with high-risk sexual behaviors. Second, large metropolitan areas also have greater numbers of intravenous drug users (IDUs), a growing risk factor for HIV infection. Third, while HIV infection and transmission are not restricted to more populated areas, those who need and seek treatment may migrate to these areas for access to medical care and social services. In many smaller communities medical care may be unavailable and financial and/or social barriers may limit access to health care services.

Declining Rates Among Men Who Have Sex With Men (MSM)

The CDC reported 41,960 new adult and adolescent AIDS cases from January through December 2000, of which 31,501 were adult and adolescent males. Of these males, 13,562 AIDS cases (43 percent) were attributable to transmission among MSM who did not also inject drugs, a slight decline from 44 percent in 1999. Since an additional 1,548 MSM (5 percent) also used intravenous drugs, it is unclear whether AIDS was acquired from sexual behavior or injected drug use. From when record-keeping began in 1981 until December 2000, men in the MSM exposure category who did not inject intravenous drugs accounted for 56 percent of all men who had acquired AIDS and 46 percent of all reported AIDS cases, a slight drop from 47 percent in 1999. Declining numbers documented in several studies have prompted some observers to conclude that AIDS among MSM has peaked.

Growing Rates Among Women

While the proportion of new AIDS cases among MSM appears to be decreasing, the proportion of newly reported cases among women is growing. While the actual number of AIDS cases in women has been declining, their proportion has been steadily increasing. Women accounted for 25 percent of adult and adolescent AIDS cases in 2000, up from 23 percent in 1998 and 1999, and 19 percent in 1995. Meanwhile, the actual number remained fairly constant from 1994 to 1997—13,887 in 1994, 13,764 in 1995, 13,767 in 1996 and 13,105 in 1997—dropping to 10,998 in 1998–99 and 10,459 in 2000. (See Table 3.5 for 2000 figures.) A far higher proportion of women than men acquired HIV through heterosexual contact. Women with a history of heterosexual contact as their only risk factor made up 38 percent of all female cases by 2000, while 8 percent of men acquired HIV via heterosexual contact.

A Decline in AIDS Due to Blood Transfusions

As a result of screening procedures for blood and blood products that began in 1985, the number of AIDS cases among adult/adolescent transfusion recipients has decreased from 664 cases in 1995, to 551 cases in 1996, to 409 cases in 1997, leveling off at 266 cases between 1998 and 1999 and 282 in 2000. The number of AIDS cases among adults and adolescents with hemophilia has also decreased. In 1996, 330 of these cases were reported; in 1997, 201 adults and adolescents with hemophilia developed AIDS; by 1999, 171 hemophiliacs developed AIDS and in 2000 only 96 adult and adolescent cases of AIDS were attributed to hemophilia. (See Table 3.5.)

Current Age and Gender Distribution

Almost all (99 percent) of the 774,467 cumulative AIDS cases reported by 2000 were among adults and adolescents. (See Table 3.5.) The remaining 1 percent

TABLE 3.3

AIDS cases and annual rates per 100,000 population, by area and age group, reported through December 2000

Area of residence	1999 No.	1999 Rate	2000 No.	2000 Rate	Cumulative totals Adults/ adolescents	Cumulative totals Children <13 years old	Cumulative totals Total
Alabama	472	10.8	483	10.9	6,198	72	6,270
Alaska	14	2.3	22	3.5	471	5	476
Arizona	876	18.3	460	9.0	7,404	39	7,443
Arkansas	194	7.6	194	7.3	2,939	38	2,977
California	5,392	16.3	4,737	14.0	119,218	608	119,826
Colorado	311	7.7	313	7.3	6,971	29	7,000
Connecticut	584	17.8	620	18.2	11,395	176	11,571
Delaware	184	24.4	221	28.2	2,558	22	2,580
District of Columbia	835	160.9	875	153.0	12,931	171	13,102
Florida	5,421	35.9	4,976	31.1	79,014	1,402	80,416
Georgia	1,680	21.6	1,237	15.1	22,626	211	22,837
Hawaii	99	8.4	115	9.5	2,445	16	2,461
Idaho	25	2.0	22	1.7	495	2	497
Illinois	1,559	12.9	1,761	14.2	24,740	269	25,009
Indiana	361	6.1	389	6.4	6,108	41	6,149
Iowa	85	3.0	94	3.2	1,307	10	1,317
Kansas	170	6.4	128	4.8	2,355	13	2,368
Kentucky	277	7.0	212	5.2	3,319	26	3,345
Louisiana	855	19.6	679	15.2	12,520	125	12,645
Maine	80	6.4	40	3.1	947	9	956
Maryland	1,522	29.4	1,465	27.7	21,390	301	21,691
Massachusetts	1,425	23.1	1,197	18.9	16,068	206	16,274
Michigan	642	6.5	767	7.7	11,215	107	11,322
Minnesota	189	4.0	185	3.8	3,741	23	3,764
Mississippi	419	15.1	431	15.2	4,411	55	4,466
Missouri	528	9.7	459	8.2	9,164	57	9,221
Montana	13	1.5	16	1.8	323	3	326
Nebraska	67	4.0	79	4.6	1,086	10	1,096
Nevada	242	13.4	286	14.3	4,393	27	4,420
New Hampshire	47	3.9	31	2.5	873	9	882
New Jersey	2,037	25.0	1,929	22.9	41,392	751	42,143
New Mexico	93	5.3	144	7.9	2,043	8	2,051
New York	7,685	42.2	6,204	32.7	139,922	2,242	142,164
North Carolina	796	10.4	696	8.6	10,320	116	10,436
North Dakota	7	1.1	3	0.5	105	1	106
Ohio	554	4.9	599	5.3	11,273	121	11,394
Oklahoma	147	4.4	352	10.2	3,761	26	3,787
Oregon	225	6.8	210	6.1	4,782	17	4,799
Pennsylvania	1,962	16.4	1,692	13.8	24,335	325	24,660
Rhode Island	107	10.8	102	9.7	2,033	21	2,054
South Carolina	956	24.6	810	20.2	9,448	79	9,527
South Dakota	16	2.2	8	1.1	162	4	166
Tennessee	755	13.8	863	15.2	8,538	52	8,590
Texas	3,151	15.7	2,667	12.8	53,607	380	53,987
Utah	154	7.2	151	6.8	1,955	21	1,976
Vermont	21	3.5	38	6.2	399	6	405
Virginia	937	13.6	891	12.6	12,919	169	13,088
Washington	359	6.2	515	8.7	9,468	35	9,503
West Virginia	68	3.8	63	3.5	1,069	9	1,078
Wisconsin	152	2.9	218	4.1	3,557	29	3,586
Wyoming	15	3.1	11	2.2	184	2	186
Subtotal	**44,765**	**16.4**	**40,660**	**14.4**	**739,897**	**8,496**	**748,393**

U.S. dependencies, possessions, and associated nations

Area of residence	1999 No.	1999 Rate	2000 No.	2000 Rate	Cumulative totals Adults/ adolescents	Cumulative totals Children <13 years old	Cumulative totals Total
Guam	10	6.6	15	9.7	48		48
Pacific Islands, U.S.				−4			4
Puerto Rico	1,244	32.0	1,349	35.4	24,495	388	24,883
Virgin Islands, U.S.	39	32.6	34	28.1	466	17	483
Total[1]	**46,143**	**16.6**	**42,156**	**14.7**	**765,559**	**8,908**	**774,467**

[1]U.S. totals presented in this report include data from the United States (50 states and the District of Columbia), and from U.S. dependencies, possessions, and independent nations in free association with the United States. Totals include 656 persons whose area of residence is unknown.

SOURCE: "Table 2. AIDS cases and annual rates per 100,000 population, by area and age group, reported through December 2000, United States," in *HIV/AIDS Surveillance Report*, vol. 12, no. 2, Centers for Disease Control and Prevention, Atlanta, GA, 2000

FIGURE 3.1

Adult and adolescent HIV infection and AIDS cases, by gender and state, reported in 2000

Male adult/adolescent HIV infection and AIDS cases reported in 2000

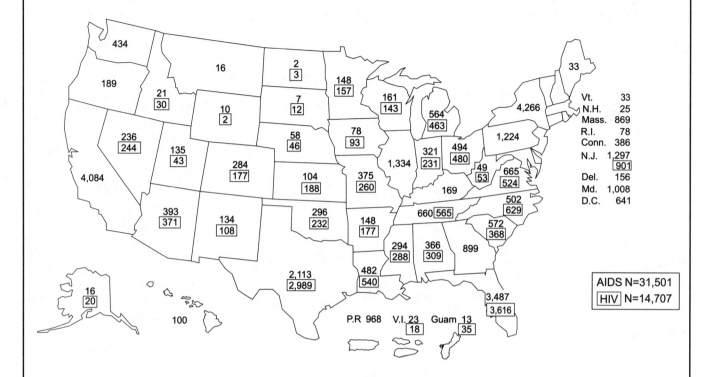

Female adult/adolescent HIV infection and AIDS cases reported in 2000

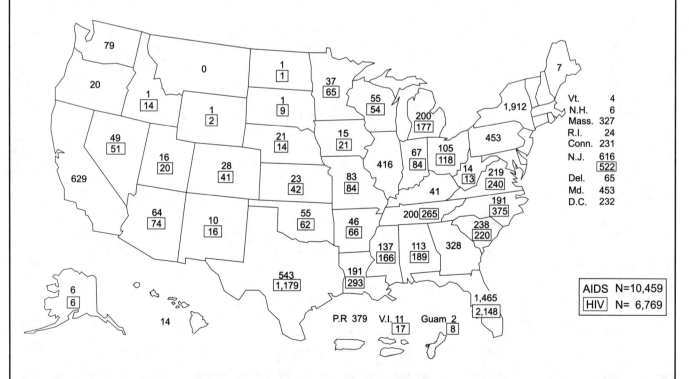

SOURCE: "Figure 3. Male adult/adolescent HIV infection and AIDS cases reported in 2000, United States" and "Figure 4. Female adult/adolescent HIV infection and AIDS cases reported in 2000, United States," in *HIV/AIDS Surveillance Report*, vol. 12, no. 2, Centers for Disease Control and Prevention, Atlanta, GA, 2000

TABLE 3.4

AIDS cases and annual rates per 100,000 population, by metropolitan area and age group, reported through December 2000

Metropolitan area of residence (with 500,000 or more population)	1999		2000		Cumulative totals		
	No.	Rate	No.	Rate	Adults/ adolescents	Children <13 years old	Total
Akron, Ohio	53	7.7	30	4.3	586	1	587
Albany-Schenectady, N.Y.	79	9.1	126	14.4	1,749	24	1,773
Albuquerque, N.Mex.	48	7.1	72	10.1	1,102	2	1,104
Allentown, Pa.	79	12.8	50	7.8	829	8	837
Ann Arbor, Mich.	27	4.8	36	6.2	399	9	408
Atlanta, Ga.	1,028	26.7	707	17.2	15,763	115	15,878
Austin, Tex.	275	24.0	180	14.4	3,868	25	3,893
Bakersfield, Calif.	90	14.0	86	13.0	1,036	8	1,044
Baltimore, Md.	1,012	40.6	973	38.1	14,306	208	14,514
Baton Rouge, La.	189	32.6	145	24.1	1,893	19	1,912
Bergen-Passaic, N.J.	248	18.5	211	15.4	5,386	82	5,468
Birmingham, Ala.	137	15.0	116	12.6	1,888	23	1,911
Boston, Mass.	1,196	20.3	1,026	16.9	14,135	182	14,317
Buffalo, N.Y.	172	15.1	83	7.1	1,814	18	1,832
Charleston, S.C.	116	21.0	116	21.1	1,551	12	1,563
Charlotte, N.C.	162	11.4	134	8.9	2,108	22	2,130
Chicago, Ill.	1,353	16.9	1,522	18.4	21,420	238	21,658
Cincinnati, Ohio	60	3.7	75	4.6	1,900	15	1,915
Cleveland, Ohio	181	8.1	168	7.5	3,330	42	3,372
Colorado Springs, Colo.	27	5.4	25	4.8	451	5	456
Columbia, S.C.	281	54.4	156	29.1	2,024	16	2,040
Columbus, Ohio	87	5.8	118	7.7	2,220	13	2,233
Dallas, Tex.	626	19.1	654	18.6	12,370	37	12,407
Dayton, Ohio	47	4.9	64	6.7	997	17	1,014
Denver, Colo.	231	11.7	229	10.9	5,536	20	5,556
Detroit, Mich.	417	9.3	551	12.4	7,736	73	7,809
El Paso, Tex.	91	13.0	78	11.5	1,072	10	1,082
Fort Lauderdale, Fla.	932	60.7	861	53.0	12,700	245	12,945
Fort Wayne, Ind.	17	3.5	25	5.0	312	3	315
Fort Worth, Tex.	133	8.2	193	11.3	3,247	26	3,273
Fresno, Calif.	65	7.4	95	10.3	1,202	14	1,216
Gary, Ind.	43	6.8	62	9.8	733	4	737
Grand Rapids, Mich.	40	3.8	36	3.3	761	4	765
Greensboro, N.C.	172	14.6	98	7.8	1,664	21	1,685
Greenville, S.C.	135	14.5	123	12.8	1,505	6	1,511
Harrisburg, Pa.	74	12.0	71	11.3	1,014	8	1,022
Hartford, Conn.	178	16.0	239	20.8	3,966	46	4,012
Honolulu, Hawaii	76	8.8	84	9.6	1,786	13	1,799
Houston, Tex.	927	23.1	693	16.6	18,956	160	19,116
Indianapolis, Ind.	183	11.9	163	10.1	2,877	17	2,894
Jacksonville, Fla.	299	28.3	289	26.3	4,419	68	4,487
Jersey City, N.J.	249	45.0	231	37.9	6,483	120	6,603
Kansas City, Mo.	200	11.4	178	10.0	3,925	15	3,940
Knoxville, Tenn.	46	6.8	45	6.5	726	6	732
Las Vegas, Nev.	205	14.8	249	15.9	3,588	26	3,614
Little Rock, Ark.	56	10.0	54	9.2	1,043	14	1,057
Los Angeles, Calif.	2,050	22.0	1,667	17.5	42,020	234	42,254
Louisville, Ky.	158	15.7	93	9.1	1,630	17	1,647
McAllen, Tex.	28	5.2	42	7.4	371	10	381
Memphis, Tenn.	327	29.6	327	28.8	3,164	18	3,182
Miami, Fla.	1,414	65.0	1,306	58.0	23,672	479	24,151
Middlesex, N.J.	113	10.0	134	11.5	3,136	69	3,205
Milwaukee, Wis.	86	5.9	136	9.1	1,962	17	1,979
Minneapolis-Saint Paul, Minn.	178	6.2	170	5.7	3,333	17	3,350
Mobile, Ala.	92	17.2	99	18.3	1,191	14	1,205
Monmouth-Ocean, N.J.	106	9.6	130	11.5	2,816	62	2,878
Nashville, Tenn.	230	19.6	340	27.6	2,736	17	2,753
Nassau-Suffolk, N.Y.	349	13.0	279	10.1	6,639	110	6,749
New Haven, Conn.	343	21.0	314	18.4	6,443	124	6,567
New Orleans, La.	415	31.8	334	25.0	6,888	67	6,955
New York, N.Y.	6,316	72.5	5,274	56.6	118,226	2,008	120,234
Newark, N.J.	914	46.8	802	39.4	16,792	325	17,117
Norfolk, Va.	272	17.4	284	18.1	3,742	63	3,805
Oakland, Calif.	345	14.7	266	11.1	7,996	43	8,039
Oklahoma City, Okla.	40	3.8	202	18.6	1,772	7	1,779
Omaha, Nebr.	44	6.3	55	7.7	756	3	759
Orange County, Calif.	261	9.5	288	10.1	5,610	35	5,645
Orlando, Fla.	441	28.7	374	22.7	5,956	81	6,037

TABLE 3.4

AIDS cases and annual rates per 100,000 population, by metropolitan area and age group, reported through December 2000 [CONTINUED]

Metropolitan area of residence (with 500,000 or more population)	1999 No.	1999 Rate	2000 No.	2000 Rate	Cumulative totals Adults/ adolescents	Cumulative totals Children <13 years old	Total
Philadelphia, Pa.	1,652	33.4	1,386	27.2	18,864	274	19,138
Phoenix, Ariz.	688	22.8	304	9.3	5,274	25	5,299
Pittsburgh, Pa.	91	3.9	106	4.5	2,357	17	2,374
Portland, Oreg.	161	8.7	173	9.0	3,869	8	3,877
Providence, R.I.	98	10.8	96	10.0	1,908	20	1,928
Raleigh-Durham, N.C.	135	12.2	148	12.5	1,996	22	2,018
Richmond, Va.	183	19.0	172	17.3	2,595	28	2,623
Riverside-San Bernardino, Calif.	378	11.8	404	12.4	6,904	56	6,960
Rochester, N.Y."	180	16.7	77	7.0	2,329	13	2,342
Sacramento, Calif."	139	8.8	171	10.5	3,206	24	3,230
Saint Louis, Mo."	304	11.8	252	9.7	4,695	39	4,734
Salt Lake City, Utah"	126	9.9	134	10.0	1,697	14	1,711
San Antonio, Tex."	202	12.9	170	10.7	3,938	28	3,966
San Diego, Calif."	547	19.4	442	15.7	10,548	54	10,602
San Francisco, Calif."	851	50.5	765	44.2	27,825	45	27,870
San Jose, Calif."	152	9.2	111	6.6	3,126	14	3,140
San Juan, P.R."	806	39.9	873	44.4	15,431	242	15,673
Sarasota, Fla."	97	17.6	131	22.2	1,450	21	1,471
Scranton, Pa."	12	2.0	19	3.0	430	4	434
Seattle, Wash."	240	10.3	301	12.5	6,662	20	6,682
Springfield, Mass."	176	29.9	147	24.2	1,729	24	1,753
Stockton, Calif."	61	10.8	37	6.6	757	13	770
Syracuse, N.Y."	82	11.2	91	12.4	1,301	10	1,311
Tacoma, Wash."	49	7.1	58	8.3	831	9	840
Tampa-Saint Petersburg, Fla.	529	23.2	470	19.6	8,334	99	8,433
Toledo, Ohio"	21	3.4	32	5.2	569	10	579
Tucson, Ariz."	113	14.1	81	9.6	1,516	10	1,526
Tulsa, Okla."	70	8.9	70	8.7	1,126	9	1,135
Vallejo, Calif."	110	21.7	64	12.3	1,378	11	1,389
Ventura, Calif."	47	6.3	43	5.7	815	3	818
Washington, D.C."	1,526	32.2	1,549	31.5	22,904	289	23,193
West Palm Beach, Fla."	458	43.6	545	48.2	7,474	205	7,679
Wichita, Kans."	63	11.5	46	8.4	729	2	731
Wilmington, Del."	152	26.6	174	29.7	2,041	15	2,056
Youngstown, Ohio"	47	8.0	18	3.0	367	—	367
Metropolitan areas with 500,000 or more population	**37,410**	**21.5**	**34,096**	**18.9**	**642,202**	**7,557**	**649,759**
Central counties	36,503	23.1	33,309	20.4	629,329	7,421	636,750
Outlying counties	907	5.7	787	4.8	12,873	136	13,009
Metropolitan areas with 50,000 to 500,000 population	**4,879**	**10.2**	**4,614**	**9.4**	**73,792**	**825**	**74,617**
Central counties	4,530	10.7	4,320	9.9	68,915	751	69,666
Outlying counties	349	6.4	294	5.3	4,877	74	4,951
Nonmetropolitan areas	**3,374**	**6.1**	**3,061**	**5.4**	**45,162**	**481**	**45,643**
Total¹	**46,143**	**16.6**	**42,156**	**14.7**	**765,559**	**8,908**	**774,467**

¹Totals include 4,448 persons whose area of residence is unknown.

SOURCE: "Table 4. AIDS cases and annual rates per 100,000 population, by metropolitan area and age group, reported through December 2000, United States," in *HIV/AIDS Surveillance Report*, vol. 12, no. 2, Centers for Disease Control and Prevention, Atlanta, GA, 2000

(8,908) of the cases were in children under the age of 13. The age difference is important because the CDC has two distinct case definitions for AIDS—one for adults and adolescents and another for children under age 13. According to the CDC, as of December 2000 AIDS had been diagnosed in more people between the ages of 30 and 39 (almost 45 percent of all cases) than in any other age categories. (See Table 3.6.)

Cumulatively, 635,451 (83 percent) of the adult and adolescent cases have been in males, and 130,104 cases

(17 percent) have been in females. (See Table 3.7 and Table 3.8.)

Race or Ethnicity and AIDS

The changing racial/ethnic profile characteristics of persons with AIDS reported from 1993 through 1999 reflects a shift in the population at risk for HIV/AIDS. Table 3.9 reveals a shift in the epidemic between 1993 and 1999, with the number of AIDS cases among blacks gaining on those of whites. In 1997 and 1998, the

TABLE 3.5

AIDS cases by group, exposure category, and sex, reported through December 2000

Adult/adolescent exposure category	Males 2000 No.	(%)	Males Cumulative total No.	(%)	Females 2000 No.	(%)	Females Cumulative total No.	(%)	Totals[1] 2000 No.	(%)	Totals[1] Cumulative total[2] No.	(%)
Men who have sex with men	13,562	(43)	355,409	(56)	—	—	—	—	13,562	(32)	355,409	(46)
Injecting drug use	5,922	(19)	140,536	(22)	2,609	(25)	52,991	(41)	8,531	(20)	193,527	(25)
Men who have sex with men and inject drugs	1,548	(5)	48,989	(8)	—	—	—	—	1,548	(4)	48,989	(6)
Hemophilia/coagulation disorder	93	(0)	4,907	(1)	3	(0)	283	(0)	96	(0)	5,190	(1)
Heterosexual contact:	2,549	(8)	29,460	(5)	3,981	(38)	52,520	(40)	6,530	(16)	81,981	(11)
Sex with injecting drug user	519		9,225		977		20,610		1,496		29,835	
Sex with bisexual male	—		—		175		3,561		175		3,561	
Sex with person with hemophilia	4		64		12		416		16		480	
Sex with transfusion recipient with HIV infection	21		417		23		601		44		1,018	
Sex with HIV-infected person, risk not specified	2,005		19,754		2,794		27,332		4,799		47,087	
Receipt of blood transfusion, blood components, or tissue[3]	144	(0)	4,971	(1)	138	(1)	3,806	(3)	282	(1)	8,777	(1)
Other/risk not reported or identified[4]	7,683	(24)	51,179	(8)	3,728	(36)	20,504	(16)	11,411	(27)	71,686	(9)
Adult/adolescent subtotal	**31,501**	**(100)**	**635,451**	**(100)**	**10,459**	**(100)**	**130,104**	**(100)**	**41,960**	**(100)**	**765,559**	**(100)**
Pediatric (<13 years old) exposure category												
Hemophilia/coagulation disorder	1	(1)	230	(5)	—	—	7	(0)	1	(1)	237	(3)
Mother with/at risk for HIV infection:[4]	80	(92)	4,030	(88)	97	(89)	4,103	(95)	177	(90)	8,133	(91)
Injecting drug use	18		1,590		22		1,582		40		3,172	
Sex with injecting drug user	8		757		12		716		20		1,473	
Sex with bisexual male	—		85		4		91		4		176	
Sex with person with hemophilia	—		17		1		16		1		33	
Sex with transfusion recipient with HIV infection	—		11		—		14		—		25	
Sex with HIV-infected person, risk not specified	25		610		29		652		54		1,262	
Receipt of blood transfusion, blood components, or tissue	1		74		1		79		2		153	
Has HIV infection, risk not specified	28		886		28		953		56		1,839	
Receipt of blood transfusion, blood components, or tissue[3]	—	—	241	(5)	2	(2)	141	(3)	2	(1)	382	(4)
Other/risk not reported or identified[5]	6	(7)	70	(2)	10	(9)	86	(2)	16	(8)	156	(2)
Pediatric subtotal	**87**	**(100)**	**4,571**	**(100)**	**109**	**(100)**	**4,337**	**(100)**	**196**	**(100)**	**8,908**	**(100)**
Total	**31,588**		**640,022**		**10,568**		**134,441**		**42,156**		**774,467**	

[1]Includes 4 persons whose sex is unknown.

[2]Includes persons known to be infected with human immunodeficiency virus type 2 (HIV-2).

[3]Forty-one adults/adolescents and 2 children developed AIDS after receiving blood screened negative for HIV antibody. Thirteen additional adults developed AIDS after receiving tissue, organs, or artificial insemination from HIV-infected donors. Four of the 13 received tissue, organs, or artificial insemination from a donor who was negative for HIV antibody at the time of donation.

[4]Thirty-three adults/adolescents are included in the exposure category who were exposed to HIV-infected blood, body fluids, or concentrated virus in health care, laboratory, or household settings, as supported by seroconversion, epidemiologic, and/or laboratory evidence. One person was infected following intentional inoculation with HIV-infected blood. Additionally, 180 persons acquired HIV infection perinatally and were diagnosed with AIDS after age 13. These 180 persons are tabulated under the adult/adolescent, not pediatric, exposure category.

[5]Includes 3 children who were exposed to HIV-infected blood as supported by seroconversion, epidemiologic, and/or laboratory evidence: 1 child was infected following intentional inoculation with HIV-infected blood and 2 children were exposed to HIV-infected blood in a household setting. Twelve of the children had sexual contact with an adult with or at high risk for HIV infection.

SOURCE: "Table 5. AIDS cases by age group, exposure category, and sex, reported through December 2000, United States," in *HIV/AIDS Surveillance Report*, vol. 12, no. 2, Centers for Disease Control and Prevention, Atlanta, GA, 2000

number of AIDS cases among blacks was greater than that of whites for the first time in the history of the U.S. AIDS epidemic. In 1999 blacks accounted for 41 per-

cent of persons estimated to be living with AIDS; whites made up 38 percent of this estimate. Hispanics in 1999 had roughly half as many of reported AIDS cases as

TABLE 3.6

AIDS cases by sex, age at diagnosis, and race/ethnicity, reported through December 2000

Male Age at diagnosis (years)	White, not Hispanic		Black, not Hispanic		Hispanic		Asian/Pacific Islander		American Indian/ Alaska Native		Total[1]	
	No.	(%)	No.	(%)	No.	(%)	No.	(%)	No.	(%)	No.	(%)
Under 5	524	(0)	2,129	(1)	768	(1)	17	(0)	12	(1)	3,454	(1)
5-12	341	(0)	475	(0)	282	(0)	10	(0)	6	(0)	1,117	(0)
13-19	874	(0)	919	(0)	523	(0)	25	(1)	22	(1)	2,366	(0)
20-24	7,761	(3)	7,160	(3)	4,297	(4)	174	(3)	81	(4)	19,499	(3)
25-29	38,283	(13)	25,564	(12)	16,507	(14)	626	(13)	334	(18)	81,411	(13)
30-34	69,614	(23)	44,093	(21)	27,268	(24)	1,085	(22)	497	(26)	142,702	(22)
35-39	69,257	(23)	48,397	(23)	25,680	(22)	1,089	(22)	425	(22)	145,053	(23)
40-44	50,497	(17)	38,662	(18)	18,124	(16)	860	(17)	281	(15)	108,580	(17)
45-49	30,632	(10)	22,833	(11)	10,206	(9)	529	(11)	119	(6)	64,411	(10)
50-54	16,650	(6)	11,778	(5)	5,442	(5)	281	(6)	54	(3)	34,258	(5)
55-59	8,923	(3)	6,420	(3)	2,989	(3)	162	(3)	34	(2)	18,557	(3)
60-64	4,916	(2)	3,510	(2)	1,649	(1)	69	(1)	18	(1)	10,174	(2)
65 or older	4,051	(1)	2,957	(1)	1,334	(1)	70	(1)	14	(1)	8,439	(1)
Male subtotal	302,323	(100)	214,898	(100)	115,069	(100)	4,997	(100)	1,897	(100)	640,022	(100)"
Female Age at diagnosis (years)												
Under 5	496	(2)	2,126	(3)	763	(3)	15	(2)	13	(3)	3,418	(3)
5-12	187	(1)	501	(1)	219	(1)	9	(1)			919	(1)
13-19	273	(1)	1,122	(1)	286	(1)	8	(1)	4	(1)	1,695	(1)
20-24	1,671	(6)	4,443	(6)	1,536	(6)	41	(6)	34	(8)	7,733	(6)
25-29	4,633	(16)	11,108	(14)	4,157	(16)	102	(14)	62	(14)	20,083	(15)
30-34	6,464	(22)	16,777	(22)	6,077	(23)	136	(19)	100	(23)	29,608	(22)
35-39	5,812	(20)	16,914	(22)	5,475	(21)	133	(18)	85	(19)	28,459	(21)
40-44	3,848	(13)	11,949	(15)	3,613	(14)	109	(15)	57	(13)	19,597	(15)
45-49	2,072	(7)	6,079	(8)	2,028	(8)	72	(10)	40	(9)	10,313	(8)
50-54	1,183	(4)	3,016	(4)	1,114	(4)	29	(4)	20	(5)	5,367	(4)
55-59	756	(3)	1,649	(2)	682	(3)	25	(3)	15	(3)	3,128	(2)
60-64	480	(2)	973	(1)	363	(1)	26	(4)	5	(1)	1,849	(1)
65 or older	959	(3)	967	(1)	312	(1)	26	(4)	4	(1)	2,272	(2)
Female subtotal	28,834	(100)	77,624	(100)	26,625	(100)	731	(100)	439	(100)	134,441	(100)
Total[2]	331,160		292,522		141,694		5,728		2,337		774,467	

[1]Includes 838 males and 187 females whose race/ethnicity is unknown.
[2]Includes 1 male whose age at diagnosis is unknown, and 4 persons whose sex is unknown.

SOURCE: "Table 7. AIDS cases by sex, age at diagnosis, and race/ethnicity, reported through December 2000, United States," in *HIV/AIDS Surveillance Report*, vol. 12, no. 2, Centers for Disease Control and Prevention, Atlanta, GA, 2000

whites or blacks. The numbers of Asian/Pacific Islanders and American Indian/Alaska Natives living with AIDS in 1999 had remained at the same rate since 1993, and were the lowest of all racial/ethnic groups in the United States. In 2000 the reported AIDS incidence rate per 100,000 adults among blacks (74) was more than nine times higher than that among whites (7.9), almost six times that of American Indians/Alaska Natives (12.7), and more than double that of Hispanics (30.4). Rates were lowest among Asians/Pacific Islanders (4.3). (See Table 3.10.)

The racial and ethnic difference is particularly alarming among children under age 13. Of reported cases in children in 2000, 58.1 percent were black and 22.5 percent Hispanic. Of those with AIDS, 91 percent of black children and 94 percent of Hispanic children had mothers who were either infected with or at risk for HIV infection. (See Table 3.11.)

HOW HIV IS TRANSMITTED

HIV can be transmitted in four ways: sexual contact with an infected person; needle-sharing among infected IV drug users (IDUs); receiving infected blood, blood products, or tissue; and perinatal transmission from an infected mother to fetus or infant.

In the United States men who have sex with men (MSM) remain the majority of HIV carriers, although prevalence among heterosexuals is on the rise. In 1987 among adult/adolescent males with AIDS, 70 percent had a single risk factor of a history of high-risk sexual

TABLE 3.7

Male adult/adolescent AIDS cases by exposure category and race/ethnicity, reported through December 2000

Exposure category	White, not Hispanic 2000 No.	(%)	Cumulative total No.	(%)	Black, not Hispanic 2000 No.	(%)	Cumulative total No.	(%)	Hispanic 2000 No.	(%)	Cumulative total No.	(%)
Men who have sex with men	7,097	(62)	223,470	(74)	3,960	(30)	78,651	(37)	2,241	(36)	48,287	(42)
Injecting drug use	1,203	(10)	28,050	(9)	3,040	(23)	71,747	(34)	1,630	(26)	40,025	(35)
Men who have sex with men and inject drugs	734	(6)	24,958	(8)	531	(4)	15,848	(7)	261	(4)	7,673	(7)
Hemophilia/coagulation disorder	71	(1)	3,793	(1)	11	(0)	571	(0)	8	(0)	437	(0)
Heterosexual contact:	378	(3)	5,586	(2)	1,587	(12)	16,993	(8)	549	(9)	6,598	(6)
Sex with injecting drug user	108		1,958		303		5,390		103		1,806	
Sex with person with hemophilia	1		31		2		21		1		11	
Sex with transfusion recipient with HIV infection	6		157		11		161		4		89	
Sex with HIV-infected person, risk not specified	263		3,440		1,271		11,421		441		4,692	
Receipt of blood transfusion, blood components, or tissue	53	(0)	3,173	(1)	64	(0)	1,077	(1)	25	(0)	592	(1)
Risk not reported or identified	1,930	(17)	12,428	(4)	4,025	(30)	27,407	(13)	1,571	(25)	10,407	(9)
Total	**11,466**	**(100)**	**301,458**	**(100)**	**13,218**	**(100)**	**212,294**	**(100)**	**6,285**	**(100)**	**114,019**	**(100)**

Exposure category	Asian/Pacific Islander 2000 No.	(%)	Cumulative total No.	(%)	American Indian/Alaska Native 2000 No.	(%)	Cumulative total No.	(%)	Cumulative totals[1] 2000 No.	(%)	Cumulative total No.	(%)
Men who have sex with men	159	(53)	3,562	(72)	72	(53)	1,067	(57)	13,562	(43)	355,409	(56)
Injecting drug use	16	(5)	258	(5)	22	(16)	296	(16)	5,922	(19)	140,536	(22)
Men who have sex with men and inject drugs	9	(3)	184	(4)	11	(8)	308	(16)	1,548	(5)	48,989	(8)
Hemophilia/coagulation disorder	3	(1)	70	(1)	—	—	30	(2)	93	(0)	4,907	(1)
Heterosexual contact:	26	(9)	198	(4)	8	(6)	54	(3)	2,549	(8)	29,460	(5)
Sex with injecting drug user	4		51		1		15		519		9,225	
Sex with person with hemophilia	—		1		—		—		4		64	
Sex with transfusion recipient with HIV infection	—		7		—		2		21		417	
Sex with HIV-infected person, risk not specified	22		139		7		37		2,005		19,754	
Receipt of blood transfusion, blood components, or tissue	1	(0)	112	(2)	1	(1)	9	(0)	144	(0)	4,971	(1)
Risk not reported or identified	86	(29)	586	(12)	21	(16)	115	(6)	7,683	(24)	51,179	(8)
Total	**300**	**(100)**	**4,970**	**(100)**	**135**	**(100)**	**1,879**	**(100)**	**31,501**	**(100)**	**635,451**	**(100)**

[1]Includes 831 men whose race/ethnicity is unknown.

SOURCE: "Table 9. Male adult/adolescent AIDS cases by exposure category and race/ethnicity, reported through December 2000, United States," in *HIV/AIDS Surveillance Report*, vol. 12, no. 2, Centers for Disease Control and Prevention, Atlanta, GA, 2000

activity; by 2000, that proportion had dropped to 56 percent. On the other hand, adult and adolescent males with a history of intravenous drug use (IDU) as their only risk factor made up 14 percent of all cases in 1987. By 2000, that proportion increased to 22 percent. (See Table 3.7.)

The proportion of adult and adolescent females with AIDS whose only risk factor was IDU has dropped from 50 percent in 1987 to 41 percent in 2000. Adult/adolescent females with a history of heterosexual contact as their only risk factor made up 38 percent of all female cases in 1997. By 2000 that proportion increased to 40 percent. (See

Table 3.8.) Researchers suggest that one reason for steadily increasing HIV infection and AIDS among heterosexuals is that an increased proportion report multiple sex partners, a risk factor for HIV infection.

Undetermined Risk

In 2000 there were 11,411 adult and adolescent cases (males and female) of AIDS with undetermined risk; that is, there was no reported history of exposure to HIV through any of the modes listed in the exposure categories. These include persons currently being investigated by local

TABLE 3.8

Female adult/adolescent AIDS cases by exposure category and race/ethnicity, reported through December 2000

Exposure category	White, not Hispanic				Black, not Hispanic				Hispanic			
	2000		Cumulative total		2000		Cumulative total		2000		Cumulative total	
	No.	(%)	No.	(%)	No.	(%)	No.	(%)	No.	(%)	No.	(%)
Injecting drug use	607	(32)	11,714	(42)	1,468	(22)	30,745	(41)	502	(27)	10,171	(40)
Hemophilia/coagulation disorder	—	—	105	(0)	2	(0)	112	(0)	—	—	55	(0)
Heterosexual contact:	678	(36)	11,280	(40)	2,449	(37)	28,608	(38)	791	(43)	12,085	(47)
Sex with injecting drug user	229		4,551		559		10,537		178		5,355	
Sex with bisexual male	51		1,507		86		1,407		29		547	
Sex with person with hemophilia	7		286		4		84		1		39	
Sex with transfusion recipient with HIV infection	11		312		8		166		3		99	
Sex with HIV-infected person, risk not specified	380		4,624		1,792		16,414		580		6,045	
Receipt of blood transfusion, blood components, or tissue	38	(2)	1,826	(6)	76	(1)	1,307	(2)	18	(1)	554	(2)
Risk not reported or identified	572	(30)	3,226	(11)	2,550	(39)	14,225	(19)	544	(29)	2,778	(11)
Total	1,895	(100)	28,151	(100)	6,545	(100)	74,997	(100)	1,855	(100)	25,643	(100)

Exposure category	Asian/Pacific Islander				American Indian/Alaska Native				Cumulative totals[1]			
	2000		Cumulative total		2000		Cumulative total		2000		Cumulative total	
	No.	(%)	No.	(%)	No.	(%)	No.	(%)	No.	(%)	No.	(%)
Injecting drug use	2	(3)	110	(16)	28	(41)	190	(45)	2,609	(25)	52,991	(41)
Hemophilia/coagulation disorder	—	—	6	(1)	1	(1)	3	(1)	3	(0)	283	(0)
Heterosexual contact:	33	(43)	346	(49)	26	(38)	157	(37)	3,981	(38)	52,520	(40)
Sex with injecting drug user	2		83		9		72		977		20,610	
Sex with bisexual male	3		71		6		23		175		3,561	
Sex with person with hemophilia	—		5		—		2		12		416	
Sex with transfusion recipient with HIV infection	1		20		—		3		23		601	
Sex with HIV-infected person, risk not specified	27		167		11		57		2,794		27,332	
Receipt of blood transfusion, blood components, or tissue	4	(5)	100	(14)	—	—	14	(3)	138	(1)	3,806	(3)
Risk not reported or identified	38	(49)	145	(21)	13	(19)	62	(15)	3,728	(36)	20,504	(16)
Total	77	(100)	707	(100)	68	(100)	426	(100)	10,459	(100)	130,104	(100)

[1]Includes 179 women whose race/ethnicity is unknown.

SOURCE: "Table 11. Female adult/adolescent AIDS cases by exposure category and race/ethnicity, reported through December 2000, United States," in *HIV/AIDS Surveillance Report*, vol. 12, no. 2, Centers for Disease Control and Prevention, Atlanta, GA, 2000

health departments, persons whose exposure history was incomplete at the time of their death, those who refused to be interviewed or whose cases were not followed up, and persons who were interviewed, had no follow-up, and therefore no exposure mode was identified. When an exposure mode is identified during follow-up, patients are reclassified into the appropriate exposure category.

MORTALITY FROM AIDS

In 1999 the average life expectancy for Americans had risen to an all-time high of 76.7 years, a figure that would have been higher, according to the CDC, were it not for AIDS, which until very recently persisted as a leading cause of death in the United States. Fifty-eight percent of all reported AIDS adult and adolescent patients and an identical percentage of all pediatric AIDS patients were reported to have died by the end of 2000. (See Table 3.12.) Nearly 100 percent of AIDS patients die within seven years of the initial diagnosis of this late stage of HIV infection. Some deaths are not reported to the CDC, or are reported as deaths from other causes, resulting in an underestimate of the case-fatality rate. The case-fatality rate is frequently used as a measure of the

TABLE 3.9

Estimated persons living with AIDS, by race, ethnicity and year, 1993–99[1]

Race/ethnicity	1993	1994	1995	Year 1996	1997	1998	1999
White, not Hispanic	80,320	86,417	91,302	98,119	106,734	114,079	121,485
Black, not Hispanic	60,655	71,818	81,152	92,167	105,142	117,110	128,941
Hispanic	31,198	36,448	40,891	46,016	51,927	57,201	62,573
Asian/Pacific Islander	1,292	1,457	1,613	1,854	2,082	2,304	2,579
American Indian/Alaska Native	573	668	723	804	888	966	1,068
Total[2]	174,244	197,060	216,010	239,382	267,311	292,286	317,368

[1]These numbers do not represent actual cases of persons living with AIDS. Rather, these numbers are point estimates of persons living with AIDS derived by subtracting the estimated cumulative number of deaths in persons with AIDS from the estimated cumulative number of persons with AIDS. Estimated AIDS cases and estimated deaths are adjusted for reporting delays, but not for incomplete reporting. Annual estimates are through the most recent year for which reliable estimates are available.
[2]Totals include estimates of persons whose race/ethnicity is unknown. Because column totals were calculated independently of the values for the sub-populations, the values in each column may not sum to the column total.

SOURCE: "Table 26. Estimated persons living with AIDS, by race/ethnicity and year, 1993 through 1999, United States[1]," in *HIV/AIDS Surveillance Report*, vol. 12, no. 2, Centers for Disease Control and Prevention, Atlanta, GA, 2000

TABLE 3.10

AIDS cases and annual rates per 100,000 population, by race/ethnicity, age group, and sex, reported in 2000

Race/ethnicity	Adults/adolescents Males No.	Rate	Females No.	Rate	Total No.	Rate	Children <13 years No.	Rate	Total No.	Rate
White, not Hispanic	11,466	14.0	1,895	2.2	13,361	7.9	31	0.1	13,392	6.6
Black, not Hispanic	13,218	107.0	6,545	45.9	19,763	74.2	127	1.7	19,890	58.1
Hispanic	6,285	47.2	1,855	13.8	8,140	30.4	33	0.3	8,173	22.5
Asian/Pacific Islander	300	7.2	77	1.7	377	4.3	3	0.1	380	3.4
American Indian/Alaska Native	135	17.3	68	8.3	203	12.7	1	0.2	204	9.8
Total[1]	31,501	28.0	10,459	8.7	41,960	18.0	196	0.4	42,156	14.7

[1]Totals include 117 persons whose race/ethnicity is unknown.

SOURCE: "Table 18. AIDS cases and annual rates per 100,000 population, by race/ethnicity, age group, and sex, reported in 2000, United States," in *HIV/AIDS Surveillance Report*, vol. 12, no. 2, Centers for Disease Control and Prevention, Atlanta, GA, 2000

severity of a disease and to estimate the probability of death among diagnosed cases. It is calculated by dividing the number of deaths from a disease by the number of cases of that disease.

Table 3.13 shows that the actual number of deaths due to AIDS increased until 1995. Since then the number of deaths has been dropping. In 1999 16,767 adults and adolescents died from AIDS, marking the lowest case-fatality rate ever. Fewer people are dying from AIDS because of more effective treatment. As fewer people become infected with HIV, the death rate in subsequent years will drop proportionally. The statistics for children under age 13 at the time of diagnosis, however, remain grim—half die before their first birthday, while the other half do not live to adolescence.

According to 2000 CDC data, 71 percent (317,010) of the males and females who have died from AIDS since the epidemic began were between 25 and 44 years of age. (See Table 3.2.) In that age group, 46,939 (15 percent) were female, and 270,070 (85 percent) were male. White and black males composed the largest group of cumulative deaths (192,276 and 121,030, respectively), with Hispanic males (64,305) and black females (37,862) ranking third and fourth.

TABLE 3.11

Pediatric AIDS cases by exposure category and race/ethnicity, reported through December 2000

Exposure category	White, not Hispanic 2000 No.	(%)	Cumulative total No.	(%)	Black, not Hispanic 2000 No.	(%)	Cumulative total No.	(%)	Hispanic 2000 No.	(%)	Cumulative total No.	(%)
Hemophilia/coagulation disorder	—	—	159	(10)	—	—	34	(1)	—	—	38	(2)
Mother with/at risk for HIV infection:	28	(90)	1,173	(76)	115	(91)	5,010	(96)	31	(94)	1,875	(92)
Injecting drug use	8		486		24		1,915		6		746	
Sex with injecting drug user	5		232		10		735		4		493	
Sex with bisexual male	1		65		1		67		2		41	
Sex with person with hemophilia	1		18		—		7		—		8	
Sex with transfusion recipient with HIV infection	—		8		—		8		—		9	
Sex with HIV-infected person, risk not specified	8		149		38		834		8		264	
Receipt of blood transfusion, blood components, or tissue	2		44		—		74		—		34	
Has HIV infection, risk not specified	3		171		42		1,370		11		280	
Receipt of blood transfusion, blood components, or tissue	—	—	189	(12)	1	(1)	89	(2)	—	—	93	(5)
Risk not reported or identified[1]	3	(10)	27	(2)	11	(9)	98	(2)	2	(6)	26	(1)
Total	31	(100)	1,548	(100)	127	(100)	5,231	(100)	33	(100)	2,032	(100)

Exposure category	Asian/Pacific Islander 2000 No.	(%)	Cumulative total No.	(%)	American Indian/Alaska Native 2000 No.	(%)	Cumulative total No.	(%)	Cumulative totals[2] 2000 No.	(%)	Cumulative total No.	(%)
Hemophilia/coagulation disorder	—	—	3	(6)	—	—	2	(6)	1	(1)	237	(3)
Mother with/at risk for HIV infection:	2	(67)	33	(65)	1	(100)	28	(90)	177	(90)	8,133	(91)
Injecting drug use	1		6		1		14		40		3,172	
Sex with injecting drug user	1		6		—		6		20		1,473	
Sex with bisexual male	—		2		—		—		4		176	
Sex with person with hemophilia	—		—		—		—		1		33	
Sex with transfusion recipient with HIV infection	—		—		—		—		—		25	
Sex with HIV-infected person, risk not specified	—		9		—		4		54		1,262	
Receipt of blood transfusion, blood components, or tissue	—		1		—		—		2		153	
Has HIV infection, risk not specified	—		9		—		4		56		1,839	
Receipt of blood transfusion, blood components, or tissue	1	(33)	11	(22)	—	—	—	—	2	(1)	382	(4)
Risk not reported or identified	—	—	4	(8)	—	—	1	(3)	16	(8)	156	(2)
Total	3	(100)	51	(100)	1	(100)	31	(100)	196	(100)	8,908	(100)

[1]Includes 3 children who were exposed to HIV-infected blood as supported by seroconversion, epidemiologic, and/or laboratory evidence: 1 child was infected following intentional inoculation with HIV-infected blood and 2 children were exposed to HIV-infected blood in a household setting. Twelve of the children had sexual contact with an adult with or at high risk for HIV infection.

[2]Includes 15 children whose race/ethnicity is unknown.

SOURCE: "Table 15. Pediatric AIDS cases by exposure category and race/ethnicity, reported through December 2000, United States," in *HIV/AIDS Surveillance Report*, vol. 12, no. 2, Centers for Disease Control and Prevention, Atlanta, GA, 2000

TABLE 3.12

AIDS cases and deaths, by year and age group, through December 2000[1]

Year	Adults/adolescents		Children <13 years old	
	Cases diagnosed during interval	Deaths occurring during interval	Cases diagnosed during interval	Deaths occurring during interval
Before 1981	92	29	8	1
1981	321	122	16	8
1982	1,168	452	31	13
1983	3,075	1,480	77	30
1984	6,243	3,470	121	52
1985	11,783	6,872	250	119
1986	19,040	11,988	339	167
1987	28,586	16,167	506	294
1988	35,481	20,883	618	321
1989	42,744	27,639	730	372
1990	48,697	31,382	814	400
1991	59,706	36,635	813	398
1992	78,646	41,197	949	426
1993	78,948	44,914	923	542
1994	72,174	49,548	814	586
1995	69,098	50,260	676	538
1996	60,216	37,049	500	426
1997	48,467	21,188	300	211
1998	40,567	17,186	217	118
1999	36,575	15,147	150	107
2000	23,932	8,867	56	44
Total[2]	**765,559**	**442,882**	**8,908**	**5,178**

[1]Persons whose vital status is unknown are included in counts of diagnosed cases, but excluded from counts of deaths. Reported deaths are not necessarily caused by HIV-related disease.
[2]Death totals include 407 adults/adolescents and 5 children known to have died, but whose dates of death are unknown.

SOURCE: "Table 21. AIDS cases and deaths, by year and age group, through December 2000, United States[1]," in *HIV/AIDS Surveillance Report*, vol. 12, no. 2, Centers for Disease Control and Prevention, Atlanta, GA, 2000

TABLE 3.13

Estimated deaths of persons with AIDS, by age group, sex, exposure category, and year of death, 1993–99[1]

Male adult/adolescent exposure category	1993	1994	1995	Year of death 1996	1997	1998	1999
Men who have sex with men	23,904	25,398	24,914	16,847	8,695	6,983	6,069
Injecting drug use	9,298	10,387	10,786	8,527	5,369	4,416	4,041
Men who have sex with men and inject drugs	3,184	3,503	3,436	2,585	1,445	1,242	1,124
Hemophilia/coagulation disorder	356	348	331	248	137	115	98
Heterosexual contact	1,591	2,010	2,388	2,108	1,473	1,214	1,230
Receipt of blood transfusion, blood components, or tissue	314	307	262	216	107	83	70
Risk not reported or identified	170	147	102	68	45	29	27
Male subtotal	**38,818**	**42,100**	**42,220**	**30,601**	**17,271**	**14,081**	**12,660**
Female adult/adolescent exposure category							
Injecting drug use	3,144	3,699	3,812	3,279	2,146	1,891	1,891
Hemophilia/coagulation disorder	17	27	30	30	21	15	16
Heterosexual contact	2,656	3,478	3,988	3,434	2,301	2,008	1,989
Receipt of blood transfusion, blood components, or tissue	239	225	234	174	94	74	73
Risk not reported or identified	76	56	56	33	20	15	19
Female subtotal	**6,132**	**7,486**	**8,119**	**6,950**	**4,582**	**4,004**	**3,989**
Pediatric (<13 years old) exposure category	544	586	539	433	218	124	119
Total[2]	**45,494**	**50,172**	**50,877**	**37,983**	**22,070**	**18,210**	**16,767**

[1]These numbers do not represent actual deaths of persons with AIDS. Rather, these numbers are point estimates adjusted for delays in the reporting of deaths and for redistribution of cases initially reported with no identified risk, but not for incomplete reporting of deaths. Annual estimates are through the most recent year for which reliable estimates are available.

[2]Because column totals were calculated independently of the values for the subpopulations, the values in each column may not sum to the column total.

SOURCE: "Table 30. Estimated deaths of persons with AIDS, by age group, sex, exposure category, and year of death, 1993 through 1999, United States," in *HIV/AIDS Surveillance Report*, vol. 12, no. 2, Centers for Disease Control and Prevention, Atlanta, GA, 2000

CHAPTER 4

POPULATIONS AT RISK

This chapter examines prevalence rates of HIV infection based on surveys of selected portions of the general population and prevalence rates of persons recognized to be in high-risk groups. The number of cases of HIV infection is likely to be higher than reported, since reporting is not universal and, as of January 2002, only 34 U.S. states and the U.S. territories of Guam and the Virgin Islands subscribe to confidential reporting practices.

INCREASE IN AIDS AMONG HETEROSEXUALS

The increase in the number and proportion of HIV/AIDS cases among heterosexuals signals a major shift in the patterns of the epidemic since the syndrome was first recognized in 1981. In 1997 the Centers for Disease Control and Prevention (CDC) reported that people diagnosed with AIDS and who acquired HIV through heterosexual transmission accounted for the largest proportional increase of all cases in 1996. During 2000, 41,960 adults and adolescents with AIDS were reported to the CDC. Sixteen percent of these new cases were people who reported that their only exposure was through heterosexual contact, up from 1985, when less than 2 percent of all AIDS cases were attributable to heterosexual transmission. (See Table 3.5 in Chapter 3.)

Between 1997 and 2000 the number of new AIDS cases dropped significantly, and the proportions of those infected in each exposure category also changed. Cases attributed to MSM represented 35 percent of all cases in 1997 and 1998, dropping to 34 percent in 1999, and 32 percent in 2000, although MSM continued to represent the largest proportion (46 percent) of cumulative AIDS cases (since AIDS was first reported in 1981). Among women, intravenous drug use (IDU) decreased somewhat from 32 percent of all exposures in 1997 to 25 percent in 2000. (See Table 3.5 in Chapter 3.) The overall incidence of AIDS based on heterosexual exposure increased slightly from 13 percent (1997) to 16 percent (2000), and the proportion of women who contracted AIDS through heterosexual contact remained constant at 38 percent.

Risks of Heterosexual Contact

Data reported through December 2000 reveal that 73 percent of adult/adolescent AIDS cases attributed to heterosexual contact resulted from sexual contact with a partner who was infected with HIV, but whose risk category was not specified. A smaller proportion (23 percent of AIDS resulting from heterosexual contact) was attributed to heterosexual contact with an intravenous drug user. Compared with 1998 to 1999 data, the number of cases reported through December 2000 that were associated with heterosexual contact with an intravenous drug user, or IDU (1,496), decreased nearly 20 percent. The number of cases attributed to heterosexual contact with an HIV-positive partner whose risk was unknown (4,799) decreased 10 percent. (See Table 3.5 in Chapter 3.)

During the 2000 reporting period, heterosexual transmission accounted for 2,448 HIV infection cases reported among women, most of whom were black (67 percent). (See Table 4.1.) Of the 1,231 cases reported among heterosexual men, 73 percent were black and 11 percent were Hispanic. (See Table 4.2.)

INTRAVENOUS DRUG USERS (IDUS)

In a 1995 report to Congress, the National Academy of Sciences concluded that "the HIV epidemic in this country is now clearly driven by infections occurring in the population of drug users, their sexual partners, and their offspring." From 1993 through 1999 the proportions of both HIV infection and AIDS deaths attributable to IDU among adults and adolescents increased; of the 14,707 men and 6,769 women reported as HIV-infected during 2000, 9 percent of men and 13 percent of women reported IDU. In 1999 IDU was the exposure category for 32 percent of male and 47 percent of female AIDS deaths.

TABLE 4.1

Female adult/adolescent HIV infection cases[1] by exposure category and race/ethnicity, from the 34 areas with confidential HIV infection reporting, reported through December 2000

Exposure category	White, not Hispanic 2000 No.	(%)	Cumulative total No.	(%)	Black, not Hispanic 2000 No.	(%)	Cumulative total No.	(%)	Hispanic 2000 No.	(%)	Cumulative total No.	(%)
Injecting drug use	323	(23)	2,394	(27)	454	(10)	4,367	(17)	64	(10)	520	(19)
Hemophilia/coagulation disorder	1	(0)	12	(0)	7	(0)	16	(0)	—	—	—	—
Heterosexual contact:	503	(36)	3,808	(43)	1,632	(36)	10,466	(41)	265	(43)	1,243	(45)
Sex with injecting drug user	115		1,212		243		2,384		52		398	
Sex with bisexual male	44		399		84		693		20		63	
Sex with person with hemophilia	6		80		7		42		20		63	
Sex with transfusion recipient with HIV infection	4		36		6		59		1		13	
Sex with HIV-infected person, risk not specified	334		2,081		1,292		7,288		192		765	
Receipt of blood transfusion, blood components, or tissue	10	(1)	138	(2)	36	(1)	259	(1)	4	(1)	25	(1)
Risk not reported or identified[2]	572	(41)	2,563	(29)	2,440	(53)	10,677	(41)	279	(46)	949	(35)
Total	**1,409**	**(100)**	**8,915**	**(100)**	**4,569**	**(100)**	**25,785**	**(100)**	**612**	**(100)**	**2,737**	**(100)**

Exposure category	Asian/Pacific Islander 2000 No.	(%)	Cumulative total No.	(%)	American Indian/Alaska Native 2000 No.	(%)	Cumulative total No.	(%)	Cumulative totals[3] 2000 No.	(%)	Cumulative total No.	(%)
Injecting drug use	2	(6)	11	(8)	11	(20)	71	(32)	855	(13)	7,383	(19)
Hemophilia/coagulation disorder	—	—	—	—	—	—	—	—	8	(0)	28	(0)
Heterosexual contact:	18	(51)	66	(49)	21	(38)	92	(41)	2,448	(36)	15,724	(41)
Sex with injecting drug user	2		11		8		42		422		4,056	
Sex with bisexual male	2		3		1		6		153		1,171	
Sex with person with hemophilia	—		—		1		2		14		129	
Sex with transfusion recipient with HIV infection	—		—		—		1		11		109	
Sex with HIV-infected person, risk not specified	14		52		11		41		1,848		10,259	
Receipt of blood transfusion, blood components, or tissue	1	(3)	3	(2)	—	—	2	(1)	51	(1)	429	(1)
Risk not reported or identified	14	(40)	56	(41)	23	(42)	57	(26)	3,407	(50)	14,590	(38)
Total	**35**	**(100)**	**136**	**(100)**	**55**	**(100)**	**222**	**(100)**	**6,769**	**(100)**	**38,154**	**(100)**

[1]Includes only persons reported with HIV infection who have not developed AIDS.
[2]For HIV infection cases, "risk not reported or identified" refers primarily to persons whose mode of exposure was not reported and who have not been followed up to determine their mode of exposure, and to a smaller number of persons who are not reported with one of the exposures listed above after follow-up.
[3]Includes 359 women whose race/ethnicity is unknown.

SOURCE: "Table 12. Female adult/adolescent HIV infection cases by exposure category and race/ethnicity, reported through December 2000, from the 34 areas with confidential HIV infection reporting," in *HIV/AIDS Surveillance Report,* vol. 12, no. 2, Centers for Disease Control and Prevention, Atlanta, GA, 2000

To offset the rise in IDU-associated HIV infection and AIDS, the Academy urged members of Congress to adequately fund needle exchange programs.

How HIV Is Transmitted Through Drug Use

HIV can be transmitted through injecting drug use when the blood of an HIV-infected drug user is transferred to a drug user who is not yet infected with HIV. This transfer occurs almost exclusively through the sharing of injecting equipment. Needles and syringes are the primary injection equipment responsible for transferring HIV-infected blood between IDUs.

There are two ways to introduce blood into the needle and syringe. The first occurs when blood is drawn from the syringe to verify that the needle is inside a vein (so the drug can be injected into the vein). The second, following the injection, is to refill the syringe several times from the vein to "wash out" any heroin, cocaine, or other drug left in the syringe after the first injection. Even the smallest amount of

TABLE 4.2

Male adult/adolescent HIV infection cases[1] by exposure category and race/ethnicity, from the 34 areas with confidential HIV infection reporting, reported through December 2000

	White, not Hispanic				Black, not Hispanic				Hispanic			
	2000		Cumulative total		2000		Cumulative total		2000		Cumulative total	
Exposure category	No.	(%)	No.	(%)	No.	(%)	No.	(%)	No.	(%)	No.	(%)
Men who have sex with men	3,458	(60)	26,135	(62)	1,814	(28)	14,023	(31)	877	(45)	3,499	(42)
Injecting drug use	416	(7)	3,557	(8)	725	(11)	7,876	(18)	207	(11)	1,552	(18)
Men who have sex with men and inject drugs	355	(6)	3,363	(8)	211	(3)	2,151	(5)	62	(3)	413	(5)
Hemophilia/coagulation disorder	16	(0)	334	(1)	3	(0)	90	(0)	4	(0)	12	(0)
Heterosexual contact:	177	(3)	1,267	(3)	898	(14)	5,174	(12)	135	(7)	578	(7)
Sex with injecting drug user	54		331		132		1,033		30		142	
Sex with person with hemophilia	1		3		1		10		—		—	
Sex with transfusion recipient with HIV infection	1		21		5		56		1		3	
Sex with HIV-infected person, risk not specified	121		912		760		4,075		104		433	
Receipt of blood transfusion, blood components, or tissue	22	(0)	185	(0)	29	(0)	182	(0)	2	(0)	25	(0)
Risk not reported or identified[2]	1,298	(23)	7,274	(17)	2,848	(44)	15,274	(34)	671	(34)	2,351	(28)
Total	**5,742**	**(100)**	**42,115**	**(100)**	**6,528**	**(100)**	**44,770**	**(100)**	**1,958**	**(100)**	**8,430**	**(100)**

	Asian/Pacific Islander				American Indian/Alaska Native				Cumulative totals[3]			
	2000		Cumulative total		2000		Cumulative total		2000		Cumulative total	
Exposure category	No.	(%)	No.	(%)	No.	(%)	No.	(%)	No.	(%)	No.	(%)
Men who have sex with men	49	(48)	210	(53)	52	(46)	327	(51)	6,302	(43)	44,467	(46)
Injecting drug use	2	(2)	18	(5)	12	(11)	79	(12)	1,367	(9)	13,142	(13)
Men who have sex with men and inject drugs	1	(1)	8	(2)	10	(9)	84	(13)	643	(4)	6,042	(6)
Hemophilia/coagulation disorder	—	—	2	(1)	—	—	1	(0)	23	(0)	442	(0)
Heterosexual contact:	2	(2)	23	(6)	11	(10)	38	(6)	1,231	(8)	7,105	(7)
Sex with injecting drug user			6		2		13		218		1,528	
Sex with person with hemophilia	—		—		—		—		2		13	
Sex with transfusion recipient with HIV infection	—		2		—		—		7		82	
Sex with HIV-infected person, risk not specified	2		15		9		25		1,004		5,482	
Receipt of blood transfusion, blood components, or tissue	1	(1)	4	(1)	—	—	1	(0)	54	(0)	401	(0)
Risk not reported or identified	47	(46)	133	(33)	28	(25)	107	(17)	5,087	(35)	26,113	(27)
Total	**102**	**(100)**	**398**	**(100)**	**113**	**(100)**	**637**	**(100)**	**14,707**	**(100)**	**97,712**	**(100)**

[1]Includes only persons reported with HIV infection who have not developed AIDS.

[2]For HIV infection cases, "risk not reported or identified" refers primarily to persons whose mode of exposure was not reported and who have not been followed up to determine their mode of exposure, and to a smaller number of persons who are not reported with one of the exposures listed above after follow-up.

[3]Includes 1,362 men whose race/ethnicity is unknown.

SOURCE: "Table 10. Male adult/adolescent HIV infection cases by exposure category and race/ethnicity, reported through December 2000, from the 34 areas with confidential HIV infection reporting," in *HIV/AIDS Surveillance Report*, vol. 12, no. 2, Centers for Disease Control and Prevention, Atlanta, GA, 2000

HIV-infected blood left in the syringe can cause the virus to be transmitted to the next user, when the next user injects drugs with the contaminated syringe and needle.

Among IDUs the risk of HIV infection is increased in proportion to the duration of injection drug use, that is, the longer the drug use, the greater the risk. Risk also increases with the frequency of needle sharing and the use of injected drugs in a geographic area, such as a large city, where there is a high prevalence of HIV infection.

General Trends

Table 3.5 (in Chapter 3) shows that 25 percent of the cumulative AIDS cases among adults and adolescents reported through December 2000 were attributable to

TABLE 4.3

AIDS cases and annual rates per 100,000 population, by race/ethnicity, age group, and sex, reported in 2000

| | Adults/adolescents | | | | | | Children <13 years | | Total | |
| | Males | | Females | | Total | | | | | |
Race/ethnicity	No.	Rate	No.	Rate	No.	Rate	No.	Rate	No.	Rate
White, not Hispanic	11,466	14.0	1,895	2.2	13,361	7.9	31	0.1	13,392	6.6
Black, not Hispanic	13,218	107.0	6,545	45.9	19,763	74.2	127	1.7	19,890	58.1
Hispanic	6,285	47.2	1,855	13.8	8,140	30.4	33	0.3	8,173	22.5
Asian/Pacific Islander	300	7.2	77	1.7	377	4.3	3	0.1	380	3.4
American Indian/Alaska Native	135	17.3	68	8.3	203	12.7	1	0.2	204	9.8
Total[1]	31,501	28.0	10,459	8.7	41,960	18.0	196	0.4	42,156	14.7

[1]Totals include 117 persons whose race/ethnicity is unknown.

SOURCE: "Table 18. AIDS cases and annual rates per 100,000 population, by race/ethnicity, age group, and sex, reported in 2000, United States," in *HIV/AIDS Surveillance Report*, vol. 12, no. 2, Centers for Disease Control and Prevention, Atlanta, GA, 2000

IDU. Another 6 percent were attributable to MSM contact in conjunction with IDU, and an additional 4 percent were attributable to sex with an IDU.

HIV is also being spread among non-IV drug users who trade sex for drugs, especially "crack" cocaine, as well as the partners of these users. Those who trade sex for drugs often engage in unprotected sex and have multiple sex partners. Persons who exchange sex for drugs and have a sexually transmitted disease that causes ulcers or sores on the genitals, such as syphilis or herpes simplex, are at higher risk for HIV infection. Drug and/or alcohol users also may be at greater risk for infection because these substances often lessen inhibitions and reduce reluctance to have unsafe, unprotected sex.

Gender and Racial/Ethnic Differences

Annual adult rates for AIDS reported in 2000 were far higher for blacks (74.2 per 100,000) and Hispanics (30.4 per 100,000) than for whites (7.9 per 100,000) and American Indians/Alaska Natives (12.7 per 100,000). The lowest rates were for Asians and Pacific Islanders (4.3 per 100,000). (See Table 4.3.)

More than 8,500 cases of AIDS reported through December 2000 were transmitted by IDUs. The number of women acquiring AIDS through IDU (2,609) was less than women who were heterosexually infected (3,981). About 19 percent of the AIDS reported in males was among IDUs, and another 5 percent (1,548 persons) were men who have sex with men and injected drugs. (See Table 3.5 in Chapter 3.)

Of the 855 women who became HIV infected through intravenous drug use during the 2000 reporting period, 53 percent were black, 38 percent were white, and 7 percent were Hispanic. IDU was more likely to be the cause of HIV infection for black and white women than for His-panic, Asian, and Pacific Islander women, who were more likely to be infected through heterosexual contact. (See Table 4.1.)

Male HIV infection through IDU was second only to men who have had sex with men as a risk factor. Of IDU-exposed men, 53 percent were black, 15 percent were Hispanic, 30 percent were white, and fewer than 1 percent were Asian/Pacific Islanders, American Indians, or Alaska Natives. (See Table 4.2.)

WOMEN AND AIDS

AIDS was the fifth-leading cause of death among U.S. women aged 25–44 in 1998 (See Table 4.4.) The proportion of women among AIDS sufferers has increased steadily, from 7 percent reported in 1985 to 23 percent reported in June 1999. During 2000, 10,459 women were diagnosed with AIDS. (See Table 3.5.)

Nearly two-thirds (58 percent) of the 130,104 cumulative cases among females were associated either directly or indirectly with IV drug use. Forty-one percent (52,991) occurred among female IDUs, and another 16 percent (20,610) were among women who reported sexual contact with male IDUs. (See Table 3.5 in Chapter 3.)

Racial/ethnic differences among HIV-infected women and their children are striking. Although black and Hispanic women make up about one-quarter of all U.S. women, they account for 75 percent of all U.S. women diagnosed with AIDS since 1981.

Women can infect their unborn children with HIV in the course of pregnancy, during delivery, or after birth by breastfeeding. The number of women who gave birth to HIV-infected babies during the years between 1992 and 1997 declined from 905 to 432. This decrease is largely attributable to the introduction of the antiretroviral drug, zidovudine (ZDV is also known as azidothymidine or AZT). A growing number of women of childbearing age are voluntarily tested for HIV perinatally (before and during pregnancy), and many women who test positive are given ZDV to prevent transmission of the disease to their unborn children. Along with antiretroviral therapy such as zidovudine to lower the mother's viral load to undetectable levels, deliveries via elective cesarean section rather than vaginal births may also help to reduce mother-to-child transmission. States with HIV case surveillance data are better able to direct resources—targeted public health education programs, health professionals, and prenatal care—aimed at eliminating prenatal (before birth) transmission of HIV.

HIV/AIDS in Women in Small Towns and Rural Areas

Most HIV/AIDS cases occur among women who live in large metropolitan areas with populations of greater than 500,000, but the number of HIV/AIDS cases is increasing in rural areas, especially through heterosexual transmission. The CDC studied five small cities/rural areas in the southern states during 1995 and 1996. All the women involved in the study had been diagnosed with HIV/AIDS. One-third (34 percent) of the women who participated in the study had never lived anywhere other than the small town in which they currently resided, while more than half (57 percent) had moved after finding out that they were infected.

A significant number of the more than 16,000 HIV-infected young women of childbearing age (15–35) live in southern states. Since a large number lived in states that do not have HIV surveillance, it is likely that there are women who have not been tested. As a result, the numbers of HIV infected women may be underestimated.

Sexually Transmitted Diseases (STDs)

Prevention, identification, and prompt treatment of sexually transmitted diseases (STDs) is vitally important for young women. Most HIV cases in young women are spread through heterosexual sex, and the increase in STDs parallels that of HIV. For instance, the geographic areas with the highest numbers of cases of syphilis and gonorrhea have the highest incidence of cases of HIV among childbearing women.

Women with STDs are more likely to get HIV because they have an increased number of HIV target cells (CD4+ T cells) present in their cervical secretions; these cells facilitate the entrance of HIV into the body. Further, women infected with STDs are more likely to shed HIV in both ulcer-forming and inflammatory genital secretions. They are also more likely to shed HIV in greater amounts than people infected with HIV alone, contributing to the spread of the infection. Therefore when STDs are treated, less HIV is shed through sexual contact, reducing the spread of HIV infection.

TABLE 4.4

Deaths and death rates for the 10 leading causes of death for females, 25–44 years of age, 1998

Rank[1]	Cause of death (Based on the Ninth Revision, International Classification of Diseases, 1975), race, sex, and age	Number[2]	Rate[2]
	All races[3], female, 25–44 years		
...	All causes	45,028	107.4
1	Malignant neoplasms, including neoplasms of lymphatic and hematopoietic tissues (140-208)	11,723	28.0
2	Accidents and adverse effects (E800-E949)	6,940	16.5
...	Motor vehicle accidents (E810-E825)	4,101	9.8
...	All other accidents and adverse effects (E800-E807,E826-E949)	2,839	6.8
3	Diseases of heart (390-398,402,404-429)	5,004	11.9
4	Suicide (E950-E959)	2,502	6.0
5	Human immunodeficiency virus infection (*042-*044)	2,149	5.1
6	Homicide and legal intervention (E960-E978)	1,922	4.6
7	Cerebrovascular diseases (430-438)	1,617	3.9
8	Chronic liver disease and cirrhosis (571)	1,206	2.9
9	Diabetes mellitus (250)	1,014	2.4
10	Pneumonia and influenza (480-487)	813	1.9
...	All other causes (Residual)	10,138	24.2

...Category not applicable.
* Figure does not meet standards of reliability or precision.
[1] Rank based on number of deaths.
[2] Figures for age not stated are included in "All ages" but not distributed among age groups.
[3] Includes races other than white and black.

SOURCE: Adapted from "Deaths and death rates for the 10 leading causes of death in specified age groups, by race and sex: United States, 1998," in *National Vital Statistics Report*, vol. 49, no. 8, National Center for Health Statistics, Hyattsville, MD, September 21, 2001

MEN WHO HAVE SEX WITH MEN (MSM)

Men who have sex with men (MSM) are still the major risk category for HIV infection, although the increase in the number of cases has slowed steadily over the past few years. Epidemiologists (public health researchers who analyze the extent and types of illnesses in a population and the factors that influence their distribution) believe that HIV/AIDS among MSM may have peaked in 1992.

As of December 2000, 44,467 adult/adolescent males whose only mode of exposure to HIV was through MSM contact made up 46 percent of the 97,712 cumulative male adult/adolescent HIV infection cases. Another 6,042 males (6 percent) had multiple modes of exposure, including homosexual/bisexual contact and IV drug use. (See Table 4.2.)

MSM contact is the overwhelming mode of exposure and transmission for white, non-Hispanic males with or without IV drug use (70 percent). White, non-Hispanic males represent almost 60 percent of all MSMs who had acquired HIV, although black and Hispanic males represented more than one-third of the males who reported same-sex contact. It is also the leading mode of exposure for black and Hispanic males; forty-seven percent of all

TABLE 4.5

Confirmed AIDS cases, 1995–1999

Percent of population with confirmed AIDS

Year	U.S. general population	State and Federal prisoners
1995	0.08%	0.51%
1996	0.09	0.54
1997	0.10	0.55
1998	0.11	0.53
1999	0.12	0.60

NOTE: The percent of the general population with confirmed AIDS in each year may be over-estimated due to delays in death reports.

SOURCE: Laura M. Maruschak, "Percent of population with confirmed AIDS," in *HIV in Prisons and Jails, 1999*, U.S. Bureau of Justice Statistics, Washington DC, July 2001

TABLE 4.6

Number of inmate deaths in state prisons, by cause, 1995 and 1999

Cause of death	Number of deaths		Rate of death per 100,000 inmates*	
	1995	**1999**	**1995**	**1999**
Total	3,133	2,933	311	240
Natural causes other than AIDS	1,569	2,179	156	178
AIDS	1,010	242	100	20
Suicide	160	169	16	14
Accident	48	44	5	4
Execution	56	98	6	8
By another person	86	56	9	5
Other/unspecified	204	145	20	12

NOTE: To calculate the rate of death, the number of inmates under State jurisdiction on June 30 of each year was used as an approximation of the average population exposed to the risk of death during the year.
*Detail may not add to total because of rounding.

SOURCE: Laura M. Maruschak, "Table 4. Number of inmate deaths in State prisons, by cause, 1995 and 1999," in *HIV in Prisons and Jails, 1999*, U.S. Bureau of Justice Statistics, Washington DC, July 2001

Hispanic males and 36 percent of all black males with HIV infection had MSM contact, with or without IV drug use. (See Table 4.2.)

PRISONERS AND AIDS

According to the Bureau of Justice Statistics (BJS), the number of HIV-positive prisoners in federal and state prisons between 1991 and 1995 grew at about the same rate as the overall prison population. Between 1995 and 1999 the number of HIV-positive prisoners grew at a slower rate (6 percent) than the overall prison population (19 percent). In 1995, however, the rate of HIV/AIDS cases reported among the U.S. prison population was over six times the rate in the general public. Though this rate of difference slowly decreased each year, by 1999 it was still five times the rate of the general public. (See Table 4.5.) At the end of 1999, 24,881 men and women in federal and state prisons were HIV-positive, but did not yet have confirmed AIDS. This represented a very slight increase from 1995 (24,256 prisoners). Slightly more than half of 1 percent of all prisoners had confirmed cases of AIDS in 1999.

Every year since 1991, AIDS-related conditions have been the second-leading cause of death for state inmates, behind "illness/natural causes." However, deaths from AIDS have decreased more than 75 percent since 1995. During 1995, 100 of every 100,000 state prisoners died of AIDS-related causes, dropping to 48 of every 100,000 in 1997 and 20 of every 100,000 in 1999. (See Table 4.6.) The sharp drop may be the result of effective treatment with protease inhibitors and combination antiretroviral therapies.

Geographic Differences

Northeastern states showed the greatest number of HIV-positive male and female inmates in 1999 (8,914 males and 1,116 females). New York had the highest num-ber (7,000) of HIV-positive inmates during 1999, both male and female (6,240 males and 760 females), representing 9.7 percent of all those in custody. New York was followed by Florida, which had the second largest number overall (2,633) and the second largest number of HIV-positive males (2,439). The third largest number of HIV-infected prisoners was in Texas (2,520), which also had the second largest number of HIV-infected female prisoners (282). All told, 2.1 percent of male inmates and 3.4 percent of female inmates in the U.S. were known to be HIV positive. In 1999, all states reported that less than 10 percent of male prisoners were HIV-positive. In three states—Nevada, the District of Columbia, and New York—between 20–30 percent of female prisoners were reported to be HIV-positive. In 1999 every state that reported had at least one HIV-positive male prisoner, but eight states had no HIV-positive female prisoners.

Testing Policies

All states, the District of Columbia, and the U.S. Bureau of Prisons have guidelines for testing inmates for HIV. Forty-four of 52 jurisdictions tested prisoners if they had HIV-related symptoms or if inmates requested tests. Thirty-eight states tested prisoners after they were involved in incidents such as fights, and 16 states tested inmates who were classified as "high-risk." Nineteen jurisdictions tested all prisoners upon admission. Three states also tested prisoners upon release. (See Table 4.7.)

HIV testing of prisoners is controversial in many states because of patient confidentiality laws requiring that medical test results be kept secret. In the state of Washington, concern for prison guards' health prompted

TABLE 4.7

Inmate testing for HIV, by jurisdiction, 1999

	All inmates			High-risk group	Upon inmate request	Clinical indication	Involvement in incident	Random sample	Court order	Other
	Entering	In custody	At release							
Federal*			•		•	•	•	•	•	
Northeast										
Connecticut				•	•	•	•		•	
Maine					•	•				
Massachusetts				•	•	•	•			
New Hampshire	•									
New Jersey										•
New York				•	•	•	•	•	•	
Pennsylvania				•	•	•	•		•	
Rhode Island	•				•	•	•	•	•	
Vermont					•	•				
Midwest										
Illinois				•	•	•	•		•	
Indiana				•	•	•	•		•	
Iowa	•				•	•			•	
Kansas					•	•			•	
Michigan	•				•	•			•	
Minnesota				•	•	•	•		•	
Missouri	•		•			•	•			
Nebraska	•					•	•			
North Dakota	•					•	•		•	
Ohio	•				•	•	•			
South Dakota				•	•	•	•		•	
Wisconsin					•		•		•	
South										
Alabama	•									•
Arkansas	•	•		•	•	•	•	•	•	
Delaware					•	•				
Dist. of Columbia					•	•	•			
Florida					•	•				
Georgia					•	•	•	•	•	•
Kentucky				•	•	•	•			
Louisiana					•	•	•			•
Maryland					•	•	•			•
Mississippi	•				•	•				
North Carolina					•	•			•	
Oklahoma	•				•	•	•		•	
South Carolina	•	•		•	•	•	•		•	•
Tennessee	•				•	•	•			•
Texas				•	•	•	•			
Virginia					•	•	•		•	
West Virginia					•	•	•			
West										
Alaska					•	•	•			
Arizona					•	•	•			
California					•	•	•			•
Colorado	•				•	•	•			
Hawaii					•	•				
Idaho	•			•	•	•				•
Montana					•	•	•		•	
Nevada	•	•	•		•	•	•			
New Mexico				•	•	•	•			
Oregon				•	•	•	•	•		
Utah	•				•	•			•	
Washington				•	•	•	•			
Wyoming	•									

*The Bureau of Prisons tests a random sample of inmates on alternate years.

SOURCE: Laura M. Maruschak, "Table 6. Circumstances under which inmates were tested for the antibody to the human immunodeficiency virus, by jurisdiction, 1999," in *HIV in Prisons and Jails, 1999*, U.S. Bureau of Justice Statistics, Washington DC, July 2001

TABLE 4.8

AIDS cases by age group, exposure category and sex, through December 2000

Adult/adolescent exposure category	Males				Females				Totals[1]			
	2000		Cumulative total		2000		Cumulative total		2000		Cumulative total[2]	
	No.	(%)	No.	(%)	No.	(%)	No.	(%)	No.	(%)	No.	(%)
Men who have sex with men	13,562	(43)	355,409	(56)	—	—	—	—	13,562	(32)	355,409	(46)
Injecting drug use	5,922	(19)	140,536	(22)	2,609	(25)	52,991	(41)	8,531	(20)	193,527	(25)
Men who have sex with men and inject drugs	1,548	(5)	48,989	(8)	—	—	—	—	1,548	(4)	48,989	(6)
Hemophilia/coagulation disorder	93	(0)	4,907	(1)	3	(0)	283	(0)	96	(0)	5,190	(1)
Heterosexual contact:	2,549	(8)	29,460	(5)	3,981	(38)	52,520	(40)	6,530	(16)	81,981	(11)
Sex with injecting drug user	519		9,225		977		20,610		1,496		29,835	
Sex with bisexual male	—		—		175		3,561		175		3,561	
Sex with person with hemophilia	4		64		12		416		16		480	
Sex with transfusion recipient with HIV infection	21		417		23		601		44		1,018	
Sex with HIV-infected person, risk not specified	2,005		19,754		2,794		27,332		4,799		47,087	
Receipt of blood transfusion, blood components, or tissue[3]	144	(0)	4,971	(1)	138	(1)	3,806	(3)	282	(1)	8,777	(1)
Other/risk not reported or identified[4]	7,683	(24)	51,179	(8)	3,728	(36)	20,504	(16)	11,411	(27)	71,686	(9)
Adult/adolescent subtotal	**31,501**	**(100)**	**635,451**	**(100)**	**10,459**	**(100)**	**130,104**	**(100)**	**41,960**	**(100)**	**765,559**	**(100)**
Pediatric (< 13 years old) exposure category												
Hemophilia/coagulation disorder	1	(1)	230	(5)	—	—	7	(0)	1	(1)	237	(3)
Mother with/at risk for HIV infection:[4]	80	(92)	4,030	(88)	97	(89)	4,103	(95)	177	(90)	8,133	(91)
Injecting drug use	18		1,590		22		1,582		40		3,172	
Sex with injecting drug user	8		757		12		716		20		1,473	
Sex with bisexual male	—		85		4		91		4		176	
Sex with person with hemophilia	—		17		1		16		1		33	
Sex with transfusion recipient with HIV infection	—		11		—		14		—		25	
Sex with HIV-infected person, risk not specified	25		610		29		652		54		1,262	
Receipt of blood transfusion, blood components, or tissue	1		74		1		79		2		153	
Has HIV infection, risk not specified	28		886		28		953		56		1,839	
Receipt of blood transfusion, blood components, or tissue[3]	—	—	241	(5)	2	(2)	141	(3)	2	(1)	382	(4)
Other/risk not reported or identified[5]	6	(7)	70	(2)	10	(9)	86	(2)	16	(8)	156	(2)
Pediatric subtotal	**87**	**(100)**	**4,571**	**(100)**	**109**	**(100)**	**4,337**	**(100)**	**196**	**(100)**	**8,908**	**(100)**
Total	**31,588**		**640,022**		**10,568**		**134,441**		**42,156**		**774,467**	

[1]Includes 4 persons whose sex is unknown.

[2]Includes persons known to be infected with human immunodeficiency virus type 2 (HIV-2).

[3]Forty-one adults/adolescents and 2 children developed AIDS after receiving blood screened negative for HIV antibody. Thirteen additional adults developed AIDS after receiving tissue, organs, or artificial insemination from HIV-infected donors. Four of the 13 received tissue, organs, or artificial insemination from a donor who was negative for HIV antibody at the time of donation.

[4]Thirty-three adults/adolescents are included in the "other" exposure category who were exposed to HIV-infected blood, body fluids, or concentrated virus in health care, laboratory, or household settings, as supported by seroconversion, epidemiologic, and/or laboratory evidence. One person was infected following intentional inoculation with HIV-infected blood. Additionally, 180 persons acquired HIV infection perinatally and were diagnosed with AIDS after age 13. These 180 persons are tabulated under the adult/adolescent, not pediatric, exposure category.

[5]Includes 3 children who were exposed to HIV-infected blood as supported by seroconversion, epidemiologic, and/or laboratory evidence: 1 child was infected following intentional inoculation with HIV-infected blood and 2 children were exposed to HIV-infected blood in a household setting. Twelve of the children had sexual contact with an adult with or at high risk for HIV infection.

SOURCE: "Table 5. AIDS cases by age group, exposure category and sex, reported through December 2000, United States," in *HIV/AIDS Surveillance Report*, Centers for Disease Control and Prevention, Atlanta, GA, vol.12, no. 2, 2000

the passage of legislation in 1996 that allows corrections workers who have been exposed to a prisoner's bodily fluids to find out if that prisoner tested positive for sexually transmitted diseases, including HIV.

In North Carolina, where inmates are not routinely tested for HIV, some lawmakers are recommending mandatory testing of all prisoners. Prison officials observe that once routine HIV testing begins, the prison system is obligated to design separate units for HIV-infected convicts. Segregating HIV-infected inmates, one official pointed out, violates confidentiality by identifying those HIV-infected prisoners, and has the potential to expose the state to lawsuits.

Drug and Needle Use Among Prisoners

While public education campaigns about the "safer" use of drugs and syringes appear to be reducing HIV infection in the general public, they seem to be having no effect in prisons, according to Reinhold Muller, a researcher for the Institute of Medical Statistics at the Free University of Berlin in Germany. In "Imprisonment: A Risk Factor for HIV Infection Counteracting Education and Prevention Programs for IVDUs" (*AIDS*, Feb. 1995) Muller noted that many incarcerated intravenous drug users (IDUs) continue to inject while in prison, often sharing needles because injection equipment is in short supply. Indeed, more than 70 percent of incarcerated IDUs reported borrowing syringes while in prison.

This is a dilemma for prisons, where syringes and needles are prohibited, as are illegal drugs, and chemicals for disinfecting needles are not readily available to prisoners. While state and federal prison officials in the U.S. want to stop the spread of HIV among inmates, most admit that they cannot keep pace with or stem the flow of illegal drugs into prisons. To minimize the spread of HIV disease in prisons, some countries such as Switzerland and the United Kingdom provide prisoners with disinfectant or clean needles. U.S. officials believe that these actions endorse illegal drug use; instead they focus on providing treatment and rehabilitation programs for drug-addicted prisoners.

HEMOPHILIACS

Hemophilia is a group of disorders in which blood does not clot properly The disorders are inherited through defective genes on the X chromosome. The most common type of hemophilia, known as Hemophilia A, is a deficiency of Factor VIII, a clotting substance. The severity of hemophilia varies depending on the level of Factor VIII present in the patient's plasma. Treatment of hemophilia involves close attention to injury prevention and periodic intravenous administration of Factor VIII concentrates, commonly known as clotting factors.

Because screening for HIV antibodies was not available until 1985, many hemophiliacs were exposed to blood and clotting factors contaminated with HIV. The high prevalence of HIV infections among persons with varying degrees of hemophilia is evenly distributed across the country, a result of the national distribution of clotting factor concentrates received before 1985. The prevalence of HIV infection differs by the type and severity of the coagulation (clotting) disorder.

By December 2000, 5,427 hemophiliacs had been diagnosed with AIDS. (See Table 4.8.) Many health officials believe that 70 to 90 percent of the 17,000 persons with hemophilia A (the more severe of the two types) are HIV-positive. The 8,000 or so persons with hemophilia B most likely have a lower prevalence rate than those with Type A because they required fewer treatments with the clotting factor and, therefore, were exposed to HIV-contaminated products on fewer occasions. The CDC cautions that Type A rates may be over-represented since the studies were performed at hemophilia treatment centers where patients with more severe hemophilia, rather than milder cases, are likely to be found.

Before 1981 most hemophiliacs died from intracranial hemorrhage; by 1995 one-third of all deaths were related to HIV infection and one-fifth were related to hemorrhage. Persons with hemophilia report that virtually everyone they know who has the inherited disorder is infected with the virus. Many wives and partners of hemophiliacs have also contracted the virus from sexual intercourse with their husbands and then, via mother-to-child transmission, passed it on to their children.

A Slow Reaction

When concentrated clotting factor, which is derived from human blood, became available in the mid-1970s, its success at stopping bleeding was so dramatic that hemophilia changed from a disease that produced intense pain, disability and the possibility of premature death to one that gave people a chance to lead nearly normal lives. Hemophiliacs could infuse clotting factors into their own veins if they felt bleeding was about to start. Patients were advised by their physicians to "infuse early and often." Each dose of clotting factor is extracted from as many as 2,000 donors.

During the late 1970s and early 1980s some clotting factor concentrates were infected with HIV. Even after the first cases of HIV/AIDS appeared in people with hemophilia and the CDC and the Hemophiliac Foundation identified this new disease as transmitted through blood, physicians did not advise their patients to alter their treatments. Dr. Donald Francis, a CDC official, recalls how reluctant some manufacturers were to remove the clotting factor from the market in the early 1980s and agrees that hemophiliacs have every right to be angry and bitter about this delay. A spokesman for the Hemophilia Foundation admits that hemophiliacs were encouraged to continue using their clotting factor because they were not sure there would be a major epidemic.

When they became infected, many hemophiliacs claim their doctors were slow to respond and supplied very little information. There was no warning to practice "safe sex" to prevent the spread of HIV. Some hemophiliacs reported receiving more information from gay men's organizations than from their own hematologists (physicians who specialize in diseases and disorders of the blood).

ANGER AND COMPENSATION. Many hemophiliacs feel they are entitled to compensation or, at the least, assistance in paying their overwhelming medical expenses. They maintain that the companies that produced the clotting factors were slow to warn the public about HIV and slow to use heat treatment to eliminate the live virus from the clotting factors (although this procedure has not gained widespread acceptance among scientists as an adequate method to inactivate HIV).

Hemophilia foundations in some countries have convinced governments or insurance companies to compensate HIV-infected hemophiliacs. Japan agreed to pay $1,500 a month to affected patients; Canada offered each patient a lump sum of $120,000; Denmark, $42,500; and Britain, $30,000 a person. France dispenses funds from its $5.5 billion pool to persons with hemophilia and HIV/AIDS. The U.S. government has no plans to compensate people with HIV/AIDS and hemophilia, and in 1995 the Supreme Court refused to hear a class action suit brought by hemophiliacs against a pharmaceutical company and other blood product manufacturers (*Barton v. American Red Cross,* 826 F.Supp. 412 and 826 F.Supp. 407. Append 43 F. 3rd 678. Certiori denied 116 S.Ct. 84). Nonetheless some companies have reached out-of-court settlements with affected persons. In May 1996, four manufacturers of blood clotting products offered $640 million to an estimated 6,000 people.

CHAPTER 5
CHILDREN, ADOLESCENTS, AND HIV/AIDS

HIV/AIDS IN CHILDREN—DIFFERENT FROM HIV/AIDS IN ADULTS

Human immunodeficiency virus (HIV) causes AIDS in both adults and children. The virus attacks and damages both adult and child immune and central nervous systems. However, the development and course of the disease differ considerably between children and adults.

Before the use of highly active antiretroviral therapy (HAART) and early treatment, there were two patterns of HIV progression among children. The first pattern, severe immunodeficiency, with serious infections or encephalopathy (a disease of the brain), develops in 15–20 percent of infected infants during the first year of life. In the second pattern, which occurs in the other 80–85 percent of infected children, the disease progresses more gradually and is similar to the development seen in adults.

Before the development of HIV nucleic acid detection tests, which detect HIV infection in nearly all infants age one month or older, the use of antibody testing made it difficult to detect HIV in infants because HIV-infected mothers may transmit antibodies alone, without the virus, to their babies. (The antibody test does not directly show HIV infection, but rather the presence of antibodies to the virus. In an adult, presence of the antibody indicates presence of HIV infection.) Infants with positive results from antibody tests at birth may later test negative, indicating that the mother transmitted the HIV antibodies to the baby, but not the virus itself.

In adults, symptoms of fully developed AIDS include the presence of opportunistic infections (OIs) and/or rare cancers that often are the cause of death. The most common diseases associated with AIDS in adults are *Pneumocystis carinii* pneumonia (PCP) and Kaposi's sarcoma, a rare skin cancer that can spread to internal organs. As many as 80 percent of adult AIDS patients have one or both of these conditions. Other disorders found in adult AIDS patients are lymphomas (lymph gland cancers), prolonged diarrhea causing severe dehydration, weight loss, and central nervous system infections that can lead to dementia.

Among infants and children, the disease is characterized by wasting syndrome, the failure to thrive, and unusually severe bacterial infections. With the exception of PCP, children with symptomatic HIV infection rarely develop the same OIs that adults contract. Though adults and children may both suffer from chronic or recurrent diarrhea, its dehydrating effect may be particularly debilitating and life-threatening to children. Instead of other symptoms common to adults, children are plagued with recurrent bacterial infections and persistent or recurrent oral thrush (fungal infection of the mouth or throat). Children may also suffer from enlarged lymph nodes, chronic pneumonia, developmental delays, and neurological abnormalities. The immune system of HIV-infected children is destroyed even as it matures.

Whether HIV-positive or not, babies born to HIV-infected mothers appear to be predisposed to a variety of heart problems. Steven Lipshultz and his colleagues at Harvard Medical School examined 414 infants born to HIV-positive women. They discovered that 12 percent of the babies suffered from abnormalities, such as defects in the heart wall and valve and reduced pumping action. These defects occur in only 0.8 percent of healthy children whose mothers are not infected with HIV. Lipshultz recognized that HIV alone did not necessarily cause these anomalies. A mother's alcohol, drug, or nutrition problems, he observed, also can interfere with fetal heart development.

A CASE DEFINITION FOR CHILDREN

Because there was limited data during the first few years of HIV's acknowledged presence in the United States, the Centers for Disease Control and Prevention

TABLE 5.1

Pediatric HIV classification[1]

Immunologic categories	Clinical categories			
	N: No signs/ symptoms	A: Mild signs/ symptoms	B:[2] Moderate signs/ symptoms	C:[2] Severe signs/ symptoms
1: No evidence of suppression	N1	A1	B1	C1
2: Evidence of moderate suppression	N2	A2	B2	C2
3: Severe suppression	N3	A3	B3	C3

[1] Children whose HIV infection status is not confirmed are classified by using the above grid with a letter E (for perinatally exposed) placed before the appropriate classification code (e.g., EN2)
[2] Both Category C and lymphoid interstitial pneumonitis in Category B are reportable to state and local health departments as acquired immunodeficiency syndrome.

SOURCE: "Table 1. Pediatric human immunodeficiency virus (HIV) Classification," in "1994 Revised Classification System for HIV Infection in Children Less Than 13 Years of Age; Official Authorized Addenda: Human Immunodeficiency Virus Infection Codes and Official Guidelines for Coding and Reporting ICD-9-CM," *Morbidity and Mortality Weekly Report: Recommendations and Reports*, Centers for Disease Control and Prevention, Atlanta, GA, vol. 43, no. RR-12, September 30, 1994

(CDC) definition of AIDS did not differentiate between adults and children until 1987, when the classification system was revised. The CDC updated the pediatric definition in 1994 and again in 1999 as more information about HIV and AIDS became available. The revisions are intended:

• To reflect the stage of disease for an HIV-infected child.

• To balance simplicity and medical accuracy in the classification process.

• To establish mutually exclusive classification categories.

As Table 5.1 shows, HIV-infected children are classified clinically by severity of symptoms and immunologically by laboratory evidence of suppression. The diagnosis and case definitions of HIV infection in children are based on a number of test results and HIV infection definition criteria in mutually exclusive categories according to three parameters: infection status, clinical status, and immunologic status. (See Table 5.2 and Table 2.3 in Chapter 2.)

As of December 1999, the diagnostic criteria for HIV infection in children 18 months old or younger require positive results from HIV nucleic acid testing; HIV p24 antigen testing for children one month or older; or isolation of HIV using viral culture. (See Table 2.3 in Chapter 2.) Prior to the availability of HIV nucleic acid detection tests, which do not rely on the detection of antibodies to detect HIV infection, cases of HIV infection in infants were difficult to accurately diagnose. This is because

TABLE 5.2

Diagnosis of human immunodeficiency virus (HIV) infection in children*

DIAGNOSIS: HIV INFECTED

a) A child <18 months of age who is known to be HIV seropositive or born to an HIV-infected mother **and:**

• has positive results on two separate determinations (excluding cord blood) from one or more of the following HIV detection tests:
– HIV culture,
–HIV polymerase chain reaction,
–HIV antigen (p24)

or

• meets criteria for acquired immunodeficiency syndrome (AIDS) diagnosis based on the 1987 AIDS surveillance case definition (10).

b) A child ≥18 months of age born to an HIV-infected mother or any child infected by blood, blood products, or other known modes of transmission (e.g., sexual contact) who:

• is HIV-antibody positive by repeatedly reactive enzyme immunoassay (EIA) and confirmatory test (e.g., Western blot or immunoflurescence assy [IFA]);

or

• meets any of the criteria in a) above.

DIAGNOSIS: PERINATALLY EXPOSED (PREFIX E)

A child who does not meet the criteria above who:

• is HIV seropositive by EIA and confirmatory test (e.g., Western blot or IFA) and is <18 months of age at the time of test:

or

• has unknown antibody status, but was born to a mother known to be infected with HIV.

DIAGNOSIS: SEROREVERTER (SR)

A child who is born to an HIV-infected mother and who:

• has been documented as HIV-antibody negative (i.e., two or more negative EIA tests performed at 6-18 months of age or one negative EIA test after 18 months of age);

and

• has had no other laboratory evidence of infection (has not had two positive viral detection tests, if performed);

and

• has not had an AIDS-defining condition.

*This definition of HIV infection replaces the definition published in the 1987 AIDS surveillance case definition (10).

SOURCE: "Box 1. Diagnosis of human immunodeficiency virus (HIV) infection in children," in "1994 Revised Classification System for HIV Infection in Children Less Than 13 Years of Age; Official Authorized Addenda: Human Immunodeficiency Virus Infection Codes and Official Guidelines for Coding and Reporting ICD-9-CM," *Morbidity and Mortality Weekly Report: Recommendations and Reports*, Centers for Disease Control and Prevention, Atlanta, GA, vol. 43, no. RR-12, September 30, 1994

using tests to identify anti-HIV antibodies, which move through the placenta into the fetus, can complicate diagnosis of HIV infection in children born to infected mothers. Almost all children born to HIV-infected mothers test positive for the HIV antibody at birth, even though only 15–30 percent are actually infected. In uninfected babies the HIV antibody usually becomes undetectable by the ninth month of life; in some babies, it may remain detectable for up to 18 months.

There are three categories of HIV-infected children: children under 18 months old who are perinatally exposed, children older than 18 months with perinatal infection, and infants and children of all ages who acquired the virus through other types of exposure.

Children Under 18 Months

The screening and confirmatory blood tests that accurately diagnose HIV in adults are not reliable for detecting HIV in children less than 18 months old because of the presence of passively acquired maternal antibodies. Early recognition of HIV infection in infants younger than 18 months is accomplished using polymerase chain reaction (PCR), a test that amplifies amounts of viral genetic material to detectable levels, HIV virus culture, or p24 antigen tests. These tests can identify 30–50 percent of infected babies at birth and almost 100 percent by 3–6 months of age. Those who are HIV-antibody positive and asymptomatic (without symptoms) without immune abnormalities have an HIV infection status that cannot be determined unless a virus culture or other antigen-detection test is positive. The test does not detect 100 percent of people who are HIV-positive. Because the relatively low sensitivity of the culture may give "false negative" results, a negative culture does not necessarily mean there is no infection. Due to false negatives, a small percentage of people infected with HIV is missed.

Infants and children who were perinatally exposed but lack one of the diagnostic criteria for HIV-infection should be observed further for HIV-related illnesses and tested at regular intervals. The U.S. Public Health Service recommends that all infants of HIV-infected mothers be given a six-week course of zidovudine therapy and that HIV-infected mothers be warned about the risks of transmission from breastfeeding. Infants with negative HIV tests at birth should be retested periodically during the first 18 months of life. Studies suggest that zidovudine therapy does not influence virologic test results and consequently, does not delay diagnosis of HIV infection.

Older Children

HIV infection in older children is defined by one or more of the following:

- Identification of the virus in the blood or tissues.

- The presence of HIV antibodies (positive screening plus confirmatory test), regardless of the presence of immunologic abnormalities or symptoms.

- Confirmation that symptoms meet the previously published CDC case definition for HIV infection.

New Treatments for Children

Prescribing drug therapy for children is often more difficult than prescribing for adults because children respond to drugs differently at different ages and because oral medication must have an acceptable taste to children so that they will take it as prescribed.

By 2001, 11 antiretroviral drugs had been approved by the FDA for pediatric HIV patients. Of these, four drugs called protease inhibitors (used alone or in combination with other drugs to combat viral infection) were available to children 2–13 years old. They are nelfinavir, ritonavir, amprenavir, and lopinavir/ritonavir. Protease inhibitors (PI) act by preventing HIV already in the host cells from reproducing.

Another group of drugs approved for pediatric use were nucleoside analogs. Nucleoside analogs limit HIV replication by incorporating themselves into a strand of DNA that causes the chain to end. These included:

- Zidovudine (ZDV or AZT), sold under the brand name Retrovir (1990)

- Didanosine (ddI), sold under the brand name Videx (1991)

- Lamivudine (3TC), sold under the brand name Epivir (1995)

- Stavudine (d4T), sold under the brand name Zerit (1996)

- Abacavir Succinate, sold under the brand name Ziagen (1998)

Non-nucleoside reverse transcriptase inhibitors (NNRTIs) comprised another group of antiretroviral drugs. Non-nucleoside reverse transcriptase inhibitors slow down the process of the enzyme that allows the virus to become a part of the infected cell's nucleus. Two NNRTIs were approved for pediatric use:

- Nevirapine, sold under the brand name Viramune (1998)

- Efavirenz, sold under the brand name Sustiva (1998)

In March 1996 the Antiviral Drugs Advisory Committee of the Food and Drug Administration (FDA) approved Videx, developed by Bristol-Myers Squibb Pharmaceuticals, for pediatric use. The approval was based on the results of two separate U.S. AIDS Clinical Trials Group (ACTG) pediatric studies (one of which was the largest controlled pediatric trial to date) and an Australian study, all of which found that Videx delayed progression of AIDS and was superior to ZDV alone. ZDV (zidovudine), which is given to children and adults, had been the only drug widely recognized to help delay the progress of HIV infection and to reduce the risk of perinatal infection.

According to Dr. Carol Baker, professor of microbiology, immunology, and pediatrics at Baylor College of

TABLE 5.3

HIV infection cases[1], by age group, exposure category, and sex, through December 2000

Adult/adolescent exposure category	Males 2000 No.	Males 2000 (%)	Males Cumulative total No.	Males Cumulative total (%)	Females 2000 No.	Females 2000 (%)	Females Cumulative total No.	Females Cumulative total (%)	Totals[2] 2000 No.	Totals[2] 2000 (%)	Totals[2] Cumulative total No.	Totals[2] Cumulative total (%)
Men who have sex with men	6,302	(43)	44,467	(46)	—	—	—	—	6,302	(29)	44,467	(33)
Injecting drug use	1,367	(9)	13,142	(13)	855	(13)	7,383	(19)	2,223	(10)	20,526	(15)
Men who have sex with men and inject drugs	643	(4)	6,042	(6)	—	—	—	—	643	(3)	6,042	(4)
Hemophilia/coagulation disorder	23	(0)	442	(0)	8	(0)	28	(0)	31	(0)	470	(0)
Heterosexual contact:	1,231	(8)	7,105	(7)	2,448	(36)	15,724	(41)	3,680	(17)	22,830	(17)
Sex with injecting drug user	218		1,528		422		4,056		640		5,584	
Sex with bisexual male	—		—		153		1,171		153		1,171	
Sex with person with hemophilia	2		13		14		129		16		142	
Sex with transfusion recipient with HIV infection	7		82		11		109		18		191	
Sex with HIV-infected person, risk not specified	1,004		5,482		1,848		10,259		2,853		15,742	
Receipt of blood transfusion, blood components, or tissue	54	(0)	401	(0)	51	(1)	429	(1)	105	(0)	830	(1)
Other/risk not reported or identified[3]	5,087	(35)	26,113	(27)	3,407	(50)	14,590	(38)	8,496	(40)	40,712	(30)
Adult/adolescent subtotal	14,707	(100)	97,712	(100)	6,769	(100)	38,154	(100)	21,480	(100)	135,877	(100)

Pediatric (< 13 years old) exposure category

	Males 2000 No.	Males 2000 (%)	Males Cumulative total No.	Males Cumulative total (%)	Females 2000 No.	Females 2000 (%)	Females Cumulative total No.	Females Cumulative total (%)	Totals 2000 No.	Totals 2000 (%)	Totals Cumulative total No.	Totals Cumulative total (%)
Hemophilia/coagulation disorder	4	(4)	98	(9)	—		1	(0)	4	(2)	99	(5)
Mother with/at risk for HIV infection:	90	(85)	878	(83)	106	(90)	982	(91)	196	(88)	1,860	(87)
Injecting drug use	21		274		20		271		41		545	
Sex with injecting drug user	9		116		10		140		19		256	
Sex with bisexual male	2		16		—		16		2		32	
Sex with person with hemophilia	—		2		2		5		2		7	
Sex with transfusion recipient with HIV infection	1		7		—		5		1		12	
Sex with HIV-infected person, risk not specified	25		195		40		248		65		443	
Receipt of blood transfusion, blood components, or tissue	—		10		1		11		1		21	
Has HIV infection, risk not specified	32		258		33		286		65		544	
Receipt of blood transfusion, blood components, or tissue	—	—	15	(1)	—	—	22	(2)	—	—	37	(2)
Risk not reported or identified[3]	12	(11)	68	(6)	12	(10)	70	(7)	24	(11)	138	(6)
Pediatric subtotal	106	(100)	1,059	(100)	118	(100)	1,075	(100)	224	(100)	2,134	(100)
Total	14,813		98,771		6,887		39,229		21,704		138,011	

[1] Includes only persons reported with HIV infection who have not developed AIDS.
[2] Includes 11 persons whose sex is unknown.
[3] For HIV infection cases, "risk not reported or identified" refers primarily to persons whose mode of exposure was not reported and who have not been followed up to determine their mode of exposure, and to a smaller number of persons who are not reported with one of the exposures listed above after follow-up.

SOURCE: "Table 6. HIV infection cases by age group, exposure category, and sex, reported through December 2000 from the 36 areas with confidential HIV infection reporting," in *HIV/AIDS Surveillance Report*, Centers for Disease Control and Prevention, Atlanta, GA, vol.12, no. 2, 2000

Medicine, Dallas, Texas, the study clearly showed that Videx alone was equally effective and safer than a combination of ZDV and Videx. Further, Videx delayed HIV progression longer than ZDV alone. Children given Videx alone and children given a combination of Videx and ZDV were less likely to experience serious infections associated with HIV or to develop other major side effects than children who received ZDV alone. In fact, the Videx and combination therapies were so much more effective than ZDV alone that the AIDS Clinical Trial Group prematurely discontinued the ZDV-only therapy portion of the study. Even in adult patients with advanced HIV infection, Videx in combination with ZDV reduced the progression of HIV/AIDS by 42 percent and, therefore, their

TABLE 5.4

Pediatric HIV infection cases[1], by exposure category and race/ethnicity, through December 2000

Exposure category	White, not Hispanic 2000 No.	(%)	Cumulative total No.	(%)	Black, not Hispanic 2000 No.	(%)	Cumulative total No.	(%)	Hispanic 2000 No.	(%)	Cumulative total No.	(%)
Hemophilia/coagulation disorder	4	(11)	73	(15)	—	—	18	(1)	—	—	5	(2)
Mother with/at risk for HIV infection:	30	(83)	362	(76)	136	(91)	1,250	(92)	27	(87)	222	(89)
Injecting drug use	5		110		31		369		4		57	
Sex with injecting drug user	6		78		10		136		3		39	
Sex with bisexual male	1		8		1		16		—		4	
Sex with person with hemophilia	2		5		—		1		—		—	
Sex with transfusion recipient with HIV infection	—		3				4		1		5	
Sex with HIV-infected person, risk not specified	12		73		40		310		11		55	
Receipt of blood transfusion, blood components, or tissue	—		8		1		11		—		2	
Has HIV infection, risk not specified	4		77		53		403		8		60	
Receipt of blood transfusion, blood components, or tissue	—	—	19	(4)	—	—	11	(1)	—	—	6	(2)
Risk not reported or identified[2]	2	(6)	22	(5)	14	(9)	82	(6)	4	(13)	17	(7)
Total	36	(100)	476	(100)	150	(100)	1,361	(100)	31	(100)	250	(100)

Exposure category	Asian/Pacific Islander 2000 No.	(%)	Cumulative total No.	(%)	American Indian/Alaska Native 2000 No.	(%)	Cumulative total No.	(%)	Cumulative totals[3] 2000 No.	(%)	Cumulative total No.	(%)
Hemophilia/coagulation disorder	—	—	2	(14)	—	—	—	—	4	(2)	99	(5)
Mother with/at risk for HIV infection:	1	(50)	8	(57)	1	(50)	9	(75)	196	(88)	1,860	(87)
Injecting drug use	—		2		1		3		41		545	
Sex with injecting drug user	—		—		—		2		19		256	
Sex with bisexual male	—		2		—		1		2		32	
Sex with person with hemophilia	—		—		—		1		2		7	
Sex with transfusion recipient with HIV infection	—		—		—		—		1		12	
Sex with HIV-infected person, risk not specified	1		3		—		—		65		443	
Receipt of blood transfusion, blood components, or tissue	—		—		—		—		1		21	
Has HIV infection, risk not specified	—		1		—		2		65		544	
Receipt of blood transfusion, blood components, or tissue	—	—	1	(7)	—	—	—	—	—	—	37	(2)
Risk not reported or identified	1	(50)	3	(21)	1	(50)	3	(25)	24	(11)	138	(6)
Total	2	(100)	14	(100)	2	(100)	12	(100)	224	(100)	2,134	(100)

[1]Includes only persons reported with HIV infection who have not developed AIDS.
[2]For HIV infection cases, "risk not reported or identified" refers primarily to persons whose mode of exposure was not reported and who have not been followed up to determine their mode of exposure, and to a smaller number of persons who are not reported with one of the exposures listed above after follow-up.
[3]Includes 21 children whose race/ethnicity is unknown.

SOURCE: "Table 16. Pediatric HIV infection cases by exposure category and race/ethnicity, reported through December 2000, from the 36 areas with confidential HIV infection reporting," in *HIV/AIDS Surveillance Report*, Centers for Disease Control and Prevention, Atlanta, GA, vol.12, no. 2, 2000

immediate risk of death. Promising as these early reports seemed, the effectiveness of Videx alone or in combination with ZDV was short-lived, because HIV susceptibility to the drugs decreased over time.

In 1999 a study conducted jointly between the United States and Uganda demonstrated that perinatal transmission of HIV from mother to child could be reduced by the drug nevirapine. The drug is given to the mother in labor and to the child within three days of birth. Initial study results showed the drug to be safe for both mother and child, and relatively inexpensive ($4.00 per mother/child dose). During 2000, the Elizabeth Glaser Pediatric AIDS Foundation, a nonprofit organization

FIGURE 5.1

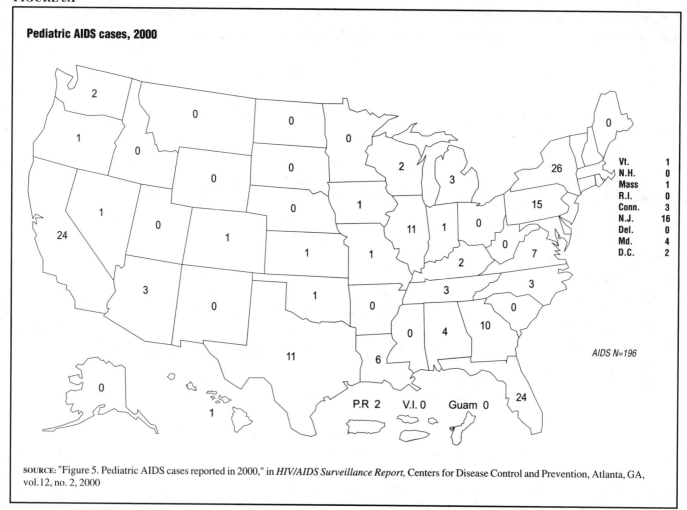

Pediatric AIDS cases, 2000

Vt.	1
N.H.	0
Mass	1
R.I.	0
Conn.	3
N.J.	16
Del.	0
Md.	4
D.C.	2

AIDS N=196

P.R 2   V.I. 0   Guam 0

SOURCE: "Figure 5. Pediatric AIDS cases reported in 2000," in *HIV/AIDS Surveillance Report,* Centers for Disease Control and Prevention, Atlanta, GA, vol.12, no. 2, 2000

dedicated to promoting and funding worldwide pediatric AIDS research, secured funds to implement this treatment in developing countries that lack health care resources and infrastructure.

HOW MANY CHILDREN ARE INFECTED?

Of the 14,813 cases of HIV infection and reported through December 2000, only 106 were diagnosed in children under 13 years of age. (See Table 5.3.) Of the more than 23,988 AIDS cases diagnosed and reported from January through December 2000, less than one-half of 1 percent (56) were children under 13 years of age. (See Table 3.12 in Chapter 3.) In 1995 the CDC estimated that 14,920 HIV-infected babies were born between 1978 and 1993. The number of HIV-infected babies born each year rose from 70 in 1978 to a peak of 1,760 in 1991. The number then declined to 1,750 in 1992 and dropped to about 500 in 1997. The CDC estimates that approximately between 6,000 and 7,000 infants every year are born to HIV-infected women in the United States. Of the 224 pediatric cases of HIV infection reported for 2000, about two-thirds were non-Hispanic black (67 percent). (See Table 5.4.)

Age at Diagnosis

In 1999 the CDC reported that more than 90 percent of children with AIDS acquired the disease perinatally and were diagnosed before they were five years old. Four percent of children were exposed through transfusions, 3 percent had hemophilia/coagulation disorders, and 2 percent had no identified or reported risk factors.

Geographic Distribution

During 2000 the reported geographic distribution of pediatric AIDS cases was very similar to that of AIDS in adults, with a high number of cases in New York, Florida, California, New Jersey and Pennsylvania. (See Figure 5.1.) The metropolitan areas of New York, Newark, Miami, and Los Angeles have felt the impact of pediatric AIDS more profoundly than any other areas.

Worldwide, HIV infection is particularly prevalent in developing countries that lack health care infrastructure, according to the Elizabeth Glaser Pediatric AIDS Foundation. The Foundation claims that such countries may have HIV infection rates among pregnant women as high as 25–40 percent. Because these women do not have access to prenatal medical care, prevention programs, and other health care, infants born to these mothers have a 15–30 percent chance of becoming HIV infected.

MEANS OF TRANSMISSION

Perinatal Infection

More than 90 percent of the cumulative total of children under age 13 who have been reported with HIV infection through 2000 were infected perinatally. Researchers have noted that the number of HIV infected infants has been declining, probably as a result of more widespread use of HAART to prevent pregnant women from passing HIV infection to their offspring. Planned Cesarean section delivery, together with timely antiviral drug therapy, further reduces the chances of mother-to-infant HIV transmission.

A number of factors have been associated with an increased risk of an HIV-positive mother passing the infection to her fetus. They include low CD4+ T cell count, high viral load (concentration of virus in the blood), advanced HIV progression, presence of a particular HIV protein (p24) in serum, and placental membrane inflammation. Intrapartum (at the time of birth) events resulting in increased exposure of the fetus to maternal blood, breastfeeding, low vitamin A levels, premature rupture of membranes, prenatal use of illicit drugs, and premature delivery also increase the risk of mother-to-fetus transmission. The risk of perinatal transmission also increases when the mother does not know she is infected until late in the course of the illness.

Factors associated with a decreased rate of HIV transmission include Cesarean section delivery, the presence of neutralizing antibodies in the mother, and zidovudine (ZDV) therapy for the mother. In 1997 the American Association for World Health reported that a 1993 study had shown that administering ZDV to HIV-infected pregnant women and to their newborn infants lowers the risk of maternal HIV transmission from 25.5 percent to 8.3 percent. The Pediatric AIDS Clinical Trials Group Protocol 076 Study Group, sponsored in part by the National Institutes of Health (NIH), conducted the study.

Caesarean Section Deliveries

In the United States and Western Europe the number of babies born with HIV infection has been reduced 50 percent by giving infected pregnant women and their newborns the drug zidovudine. Before widespread use of zidovudine, about 500 American babies per year, nearly all of them African American and Hispanic, were infected with HIV from their mothers. By 2000, there were only 224 reported cases of maternal-to-child transmission in the United States. Worldwide, 9,000 babies are born annually that are infected with HIV. Infection usually occurs during the last stages of pregnancy, most often during labor and delivery. French researcher Dr. Laurent Mandelbrot of the Cochin-Port Royal Hospital in Paris, France, reported in "Perinatal HIV-1 Transmission: Interaction Between Zidovudine Prophylaxis and Mode of Delivery in the French Perinatal Cohort" (*The Journal of the American Medical Association*, vol. 280, no. 1, 1998) that planned Cesarean delivery, together with the standard ZDV treatment, may prevent more cases of mother-to-baby HIV infection.

Some Children Beat the Virus

Marie-Louise Newell and colleagues, in the *European Collaborative Study* ("Detection of Virus in Vertically Exposed HIV-Antibody-Negative Children," *The Lancet*, Vol. 347, January 27, 1996), found that some children who acquired HIV perinatally later beat the infection. From May 1985 to August 1994, 299 children born to HIV-positive mothers were tested every three months from birth to 18 months of age. Of the 299 babies, 35 tested negative for the HIV antibody at birth, while 255 tested negative after first testing positive.

The remaining nine were found to be HIV-positive, even after several tests. Eventually, however, they tested negative for the HIV antibody also. All nine had been bottle-fed only, and eight had been delivered vaginally. Six of the nine babies were consistently negative even after having tested positive on more than one occasion, while three were intermittently HIV-positive. The *European Collaborative Study* also found that the three children in whom HIV was detected intermittently developed immunological tolerance at older ages or somehow separated the virus, placing it in lymphatic (located in the lymph nodes) tissue, where it remained dormant. These three children are permanently classified as HIV-negative.

To date, scientists do not know the mechanism that triggers this reversal. Interest in persons who convert from HIV-positive is high because by identifying the mechanism by which HIV-positive infants clear the virus may help to develop more effective treatments including immunization against HIV infection.

Gene Mutation in Some Babies May Help

A gene mutation that slows the progress of HIV in adults was shown in the late 1990s to help HIV-infected newborns avoid serious AIDS-associated illnesses longer than babies who do not have the mutation. The gene, called CCR5, is present in 10–15 percent of whites, but is not found in Asians or blacks. Researchers hope that further investigation of the CCR5 gene will eventually help them to develop drugs to prevent or destroy HIV in newborns.

HIV-Positive Mothers Having Babies

Many HIV-positive women who have babies are not aware of their HIV status. Even when pregnant women learn that they are HIV-positive, they often decide to continue the pregnancy despite the risk of passing the infection to their children. Some women choose to become pregnant

TABLE 5.5

HIV infection cases[1] by sex, age at diagnosis, and race/ethnicity, through December 2000

Male Age at diagnosis (years)	White, not Hispanic		Black, not Hispanic		Hispanic		Asian/Pacific Islander		American Indian/ Alaska Native		Total[2]	
	No.	(%)	No.	(%)	No.	(%)	No.	(%)	No.	(%)	No.	(%)
Under 5	170	(0)	525	(1)	89	(1)	4	(1)	2	(0)	794	(1)
5–12	99	(0)	117	(0)	40	(0)	3	(1)			265	(0)
13–19	814	(2)	1,398	(3)	150	(2)	9	(2)	17	(3)	2,412	(2)
20–24	5,196	(12)	5,471	(12)	987	(12)	57	(14)	113	(18)	11,951	(12)
25–29	9,278	(22)	7,866	(17)	1,806	(21)	89	(22)	156	(24)	19,468	(20)
30–34	9,912	(23)	9,317	(21)	1,978	(23)	115	(28)	140	(22)	21,759	(22)
35–39	7,670	(18)	8,404	(19)	1,637	(19)	52	(13)	104	(16)	18,125	(18)
40–44	4,547	(11)	5,934	(13)	917	(11)	39	(10)	57	(9)	11,672	(12)
45–49	2,361	(6)	3,273	(7)	496	(6)	18	(4)	25	(4)	6,280	(6)
50–54	1,243	(3)	1,546	(3)	227	(3)	10	(2)	12	(2)	3,092	(3)
55–59	528	(1)	797	(2)	111	(1)	4	(1)	8	(1)	1,469	(1)
60–64	298	(1)	388	(1)	63	(1)	2	(0)	3	(0)	765	(1)
65 or older	268	(1)	376	(1)	58	(1)	3	(1)	2	(0)	719	(1)
Male subtotal	**42,384**	**(100)**	**45,412**	**(100)**	**8,559**	**(100)**	**405**	**(100)**	**639**	**(100)**	**98,771**	**(100)**
Female **Age at diagnosis (years)**												
Under 5	163	(2)	588	(2)	89	(3)	5	(3)	8	(3)	860	(2)
5–12	44	(0)	131	(0)	32	(1)	2	(1)	2	(1)	215	(1)
13–19	628	(7)	2,320	(9)	172	(6)	7	(5)	21	(9)	3,167	(8)
20–24	1,561	(17)	4,284	(16)	428	(15)	36	(25)	42	(18)	6,407	(16)
25–29	1,834	(20)	4,985	(19)	570	(20)	35	(24)	38	(16)	7,527	(19)
30–34	1,782	(20)	4,982	(19)	591	(21)	23	(16)	41	(18)	7,500	(19)
35–39	1,412	(15)	3,961	(15)	396	(14)	13	(9)	42	(18)	5,881	(15)
40–44	775	(8)	2,587	(10)	249	(9)	11	(8)	27	(12)	3,688	(9)
45–49	467	(5)	1,314	(5)	167	(6)	5	(3)	9	(4)	1,985	(5)
50–54	208	(2)	637	(2)	75	(3)	2	(1)	1	(0)	930	(2)
55–59	111	(1)	338	(1)	49	(2)	2	(1)	—	—	509	(1)
60–64	50	(1)	185	(1)	24	(1)	—	—	1	(0)	260	(1)
65 or older	87	(1)	192	(1)	16	(1)	2	(1)	—	—	300	(1)
Female subtotal	**9,122**	**(100)**	**26,504**	**(100)**	**2,858**	**(100)**	**143**	**(100)**	**232**	**(100)**	**39,229**	**(100)**
Total[3]	**51,507**		**71,920**		**11,417**		**548**		**871**		**138,011**	

[1] Includes only persons reported with HIV infection who have not developed AIDS.
[2] Includes 1,372 males, 370 females, and 6 persons of unknown sex whose race/ethnicity is unknown.
[3] Includes 11 persons whose sex is unknown.

SOURCE: "Table 8. HIV infection cases by sex, age at diagnosis, and race/ethnicity, reported through December 2000, from the 36 areas with confidential HIV infection reporting," in *HIV/AIDS Surveillance Report,* Centers for Disease Control and Prevention, Atlanta, GA, vol.12, no. 2, 2000

already knowing that they are HIV-infected. Many people consider HIV-positive women who decide to have babies as selfish and unconcerned with the potentially frightening consequences of their actions. Still others regard the decision as strictly personal and understandable. Their choice reflects an optimism that is fostered by effective drug therapies and a new reality—many people with HIV infection are living longer, more comfortably, and asymptomatically.

The choice to bear children also reflects societal and environmental realities, as well as attitudes about death and illness. Most women with HIV/AIDS live in poverty; they do not have easy access to medical care, and socioeconomic problems such as violence, homelessness, separated families, and low literacy rates challenge children's chances of leading long, safe, and healthy lives. Tracie M. Gardner, an AIDS policy analyst for the Federation of Protestant Welfare Agencies, believes that for many women in poor communities, HIV infection is the least of

their problems. Gardner tells the story of a pregnant inner-city woman in her early twenties who, when told she was HIV infected and had ten years to live, replied that this was nine more years than she thought she had.

Regardless of socioeconomic background, many HIV-infected women feel that the decision to have children is intensely personal and should not be questioned. Said one such woman, "I see mothers screaming and berating and hitting their kids. Should legislation be passed preventing them from having kids? And what if my baby only lives five years? Who's to say that because it's a shorter life it was not a life worth living?"

LIVING LONG ENOUGH TO KNOW

Surviving into Their Teens

When children who are now 15–17 years old were born, relatively little was known about HIV/AIDS. Officials at the CDC report that most children infected from birth now survive beyond age five. In 2000 an estimated 2,703 children in the United States were living with AIDS, and another 2,134 children up to age twelve were HIV-positive but had not yet developed AIDS. (See Table 5.5.) While many HIV infected children die as infants and toddlers, it is not uncommon for others to reach their teens.

Medical experts have distinguished three distinct patterns of disease progression among HIV-infected children. The first group consists of about one-fourth of infected children who show symptoms within their first 18 months. For these children, despite treatment, progression to AIDS is more rapid than for the other two groups. The children in the second group experience a less aggressive progression and often have milder or briefer spells of symptoms, often living to be about 3–5 years old. The third group is a recently emerging group of survivors. These children have grown up with few, if any, symptoms. Some were not diagnosed until they were 9–11 years old. From New York City, where more than one-fifth of the nation's pediatric AIDS cases reside, there are reports of children as old as 14 years who were infected at birth but remained asymptomatic and undiagnosed.

Dealing with Physical and Emotional Problems

When HIV-infected children died in the early years of the AIDS epidemic, they were generally unaware of what was happening to them. Today, at the Children's Evaluation and Rehabilitation Center of the Albert Einstein College of Medicine's Rose Kennedy Center in the Bronx, school-aged children meet with social workers in a support group to handle the physical and emotional ordeals of growing up with HIV and AIDS. These children are part of an increasing number born with HIV who have survived long enough to realize what it means. They must learn to cope with the physical, psychological, and emotional consequences of HIV/AIDS.

The children deal with problems unique to their situations—a mother's death from AIDS, keeping their disease a secret from classmates at school, the fear of dying, and coping with the deaths of members of their support group. Other concerns range from the dread of having their teeth pulled (because they decay unusually quickly) to the taunting the children receive at school because they may be short and underweight. Discussions range from what heaven is like to practical advice about taking ZDV in capsules rather than the bitter liquid form. When asked by a visitor what he wanted to be when he grew up, one child responded, "I never think about it."

One More Problem

Many children do not know that they are HIV-positive. In some cases their parents or foster parents have tried to protect them and do not want them to know. Others fear that the children will not be able to keep the news from other children, teachers, and neighbors. Some parents do not tell their children for fear the children will blame them for passing on the infection. Just as poignantly, many that know keep their illness a secret even from their siblings. For those who know of their condition, HIV/AIDS is one more hardship in a life often made difficult by poverty, instability, and the loss of loved ones—especially parents. A child whose mother died from AIDS when he was five years old was understandably bitter about the fact that he was the only one of three siblings to be infected.

WHO WILL CARE FOR THEM?

The HIV/AIDS epidemic has created many tragedies, including millions of orphans. The World Health Organization (WHO) in Geneva, Switzerland, estimated that by the end of 2000, there were more than 13 million children worldwide orphaned by parents who died of AIDS. According to U.S. experts, 40 million children worldwide will lose one or both parents to AIDS between 1997 and 2010. In Africa alone, during 1999, there were more than 8 million AIDS orphans and 1 million HIV-positive children.

It is not always possible to find someone to care for an orphan of parents who died of AIDS, particularly if the orphan also has HIV or AIDS. Some family members may be hesitant to take in the orphan for fear the child may spread the infection. In a growing number of cases, however, grandparents (in most cases, grandmothers) are taking these orphans into their homes. This may be a burden on older people who have lost their own children and may feel too old, tired, or impoverished to rear another family. They also may fear that they will die before their grandchildren do, leaving no one to care for them. It is no less difficult for the children who have lost their parents and fear they will probably miss the advantages they would have had with younger parents, such as being able to play more active childhood games.

Older orphans struggle with the rage, shame, and isolation of losing a parent to AIDS. Observers are finding that the AIDS epidemic is creating a class of particularly troubled youth. All children who lose a parent suffer to some degree, but for those whose parents died from AIDS, embarrassment and secrecy often compound the trauma. Teens whose parents became infected as a result of injecting drugs or unsafe sex are often torn between feeling sorry for their parents and blaming them for their illnesses.

ADOLESCENTS, YOUNG ADULTS, AND HIV/AIDS

In 2000 the number of AIDS cases among adolescents was comparatively low. As of December 2000 the CDC reported 4,061 cumulative (since reporting began in 1981)

TABLE 5.6

HIV infection cases[1] in adolescents and adults under age 25, by sex and exposure category, through December 2000

| | 13-19 years old | | | | 20-24 years old | | | |
| | 2000 | | Cumulative total | | 2000 | | Cumulative total | |
Male exposure category	No.	(%)	No.	(%)	No.	(%)	No.	(%)
Men who have sex with men	203	(59)	1,246	(52)	758	(53)	6,691	(56)
Injecting drug use	7	(2)	110	(5)	64	(4)	674	(6)
Men who have sex with men and inject drugs	12	(3)	115	(5)	71	(5)	795	(7)
Hemophilia/coagulation disorder	3	(1)	106	(4)	7	(0)	85	(1)
Heterosexual contact:	12	(3)	164	(7)	100	(7)	784	(7)
Sex with injecting drug user	1		26		7		108	
Sex with person with hemophilia	—		2		—		—	
Sex with transfusion recipient with HIV infection	—		—		—		7	
Sex with HIV-infected person, risk not specified	11		136		93		669	
Receipt of blood transfusion, blood components, or tissue	—	—	12	(0)	2	(0)	28	(0)
Risk not reported or identified[2]	110	(32)	659	(27)	435	(30)	2,894	(24)
Male subtotal	**347**	**(100)**	**2,412**	**(100)**	**1,437**	**(100)**	**11,951**	**(100)**
Female exposure category								
Injecting drug use	25	(5)	232	(7)	93	(9)	770	(12)
Hemophilia/coagulation disorder	—	—	—	—	1	(0)	5	(0)
Heterosexual contact:	201	(38)	1,544	(49)	403	(38)	2,947	(46)
Sex with injecting drug user	21		257		40		628	
Sex with bisexual male	12		112		27		240	
Sex with person with hemophilia	2		22		4		40	
Sex with transfusion recipient with HIV infection	—		4		1		18	
Sex with HIV-infected person, risk not specified	166		1,149		331		2,021	
Receipt of blood transfusion, blood components, or tissue	3	(1)	20	(1)	5	(0)	30	(0)
Risk not reported or identified	303	(57)	1,371	(43)	555	(53)	2,655	(41)
Female subtotal	**532**	**(100)**	**3,167**	**(100)**	**1,057**	**(100)**	**6,407**	**(100)**
Total[3]	879		5,580		2,496		18,360	

[1]Includes only persons reported with HIV infection who have not developed AIDS.
[2]For HIV infection cases, "risk not reported or identified" refers primarily to persons whose mode of exposure was not reported and who have not been followed up to determine their mode of exposure, and to a smaller number of persons who are not reported with one of the exposures listed above after follow-up.
[3]Includes 3 persons whose sex is unknown.

SOURCE: "Table 14. HIV infection cases in adolescents and adults under age 25, by sex and exposure category, reported through December 2000, from the 34 areas with confidential HIV infection reporting," in *HIV/AIDS Surveillance Report*, Centers for Disease Control and Prevention, Atlanta, GA, vol.12, no. 2, 2000

cases among 13- to 19-year-olds, about 0.5 percent of the total 774,467 cases reported—a proportion that has remained basically unchanged for 12 years. (See Table 3.6 in Chapter 3.) Approximately one in five reported AIDS cases is diagnosed in a person in the 20–29 age group. However, since the period between the time of infection and onset of symptoms is about 10 years, it is highly probable that many of those in their early twenties became infected as teenagers. In addition during 2000 nearly 900 cases of HIV infection were reported among adolescents 13–19 years old. (See Table 5.6.) Most HIV infection and AIDS cases reported among teens were clustered in New York and Florida.

Patterns of Infection

The transmission and course of HIV infection among adolescents and adults follow similar patterns. Male adolescents are infected primarily as a result of MSM activity (52 percent) and through unidentified exposure (27 percent). Almost all female adolescents with AIDS became infected through unidentified activity (43 percent) or heterosexual contact (49 percent); another 7 percent became infected from IDU. Ten percent of male adolescents were infected through IDU alone or through homosexual activity as well as intravenous drug use. (See Table 5.6.)

Minorities are disproportionately affected by HIV. By December 2000, 58 percent of males between the ages of 13 and 19 diagnosed with HIV infection were black and 6.2 percent were Hispanic. (See Table 5.5.) Seventy-three percent of all 13- to 19-year-old females with HIV were black, while 5.4 percent were Hispanic.

Though females between the ages 13 and 19 were more likely than males to be diagnosed with HIV in 2000 (3,167 females and 2,412 males), this trend ends after age 19. Far more young people were diagnosed when they reached 20–24 years of age, and in this age group, almost twice as many males as females were diagnosed with HIV (11,951 and 6,407, respectively). (See Table 5.5.)

The characteristics of adolescence—a time of development, uncertainty, and a misleading sense of bravado and immortality, often combined with pushing the boundaries of good sense—create the potential for some young people to become particularly vulnerable to HIV infection. For many, this is a time of experimentation and risk-taking, often in terms of sexual behavior or use of alcohol and illicit drugs. Some adolescents, struggling with their sexuality, may engage in homosexual encounters away from home but maintain and engage in heterosexual relationships in their neighborhoods to avoid suspicion.

CLINICS FOR HOMELESS AND RUNAWAY YOUTH. In the early 1990s the CDC conducted anonymous surveys to gather information about risk behavior. Despite the anonymity of the surveys, the prevalence of certain risk behaviors, such as MSM contact and IDU, were probably underreported because most teens are reluctant to admit to such behaviors. Nonetheless the prevalence of recorded HIV risks was quite high.

From 4 to 28 percent of all male clients at four clinics for homeless and runaway youth had a history of MSM contact. This risk behavior accounted for 25–95 percent of all HIV infections among men at each clinic. Heterosexual women without a history of intravenous drug use accounted for 66–100 percent of the HIV infections among women, implying that infection came from contact with infected partners. Surprisingly, IDU was responsible for few HIV infections; fewer than 2 percent of clients at three clinics and 17 percent at one clinic reported IDU. In general, only 6 of the 103 (6 percent) HIV-positive clients at the four clinics that conducted the risk surveys reported injecting drugs.

Most Adolescents Are Sexually Active

Even though the growth in the rate of HIV/AIDS has slowed in the United States, the rate among young Americans continues to rise. Most HIV cases among youth have been spread sexually. Approximately three-fourths of adolescents who become infected with HIV are heterosexual females and adolescent males who engage in MSM.

Adolescents are having sex more frequently and earlier than ever before. In 1968, 35 percent of teenage females and 55 percent of teenage males reported that they had had sexual intercourse before the age of 18. According to the CDC, in 1999, 11.7 percent of ninth graders reported that they had had sexual intercourse before the age of 13, and 38.6 percent of them had had sexual intercourse by the ninth grade. In 1999, 65 percent of high school seniors reported that they have had sexual intercourse.

SEXUALLY TRANSMITTED DISEASES (STDS). Teenagers engaging in sexual activity before becoming sufficiently mature, together with ineffective contraceptive methods, have led to record high rates of sexually transmitted diseases (STDs) among heterosexuals of all age groups. Of the estimated 12 million new cases of STDs in the United States each year, 3 million (25 percent) occur among teenagers 13–19 years old. According to the CDC, about one in five Americans 12 years old and older has an STD; most in this group are unaware they are infected.

Although overall rates of infection for some STDs, such as gonorrhea, declined during the 1990s, gonorrhea infections among African Americans increased by more than 5 percent from 1997 to 1999, and infection with genital herpes also increased. A CDC publication *Tracking the Hidden Epidemics: Trends in STDs in the United States* reported gonorrhea infection rates among African Americans 30 times higher than for whites. More than one in five Americans is estimated to have genital herpes infection, and African American women, especially those aged 15–19 years old, are at high risk for infection with genital herpes. Recent studies and health education programs have focused on teaching African American teens aged 14–18 about the relationship between consistent condom use and the prevention of STDs. Condoms are however, less effective in halting the spread of genital herpes than other STDs because herpes may be transmitted from parts of the body not covered by a condom.

Behaviors That Increase Risk

American teens often engage in behaviors that can put them at risk for acquiring HIV infection. As described earlier, not only are more than half of all high school students sexually active by the time they graduate, but about one-fourth (23 percent) also reported having had sex with four or more partners. Among sexually active students, fewer than half (46 percent) had used a latex condom during their last sexual intercourse. Between 1985 and 1995, while the proportion of high schools teaching students about condom use rose 59 percent, condom use among high school students increased only 17 percent.

Hemophilia-Associated HIV/AIDS

From 1982, when the first cases of HIV/AIDS in hemophiliacs were reported, through December 2000,

106 cases of the 5,579 teens with HIV infection involved teens with hemophilia (a hereditary disease in which the blood lacks normal clotting factors).(See Table 5.6.) While females pass the hemophilia gene from generation to generation, the vast majority of these women do not have hemophilia; they simply carry the gene. Through December 2000 adolescent hemophiliacs made up about 14 percent of the 5,427 hemophilia-associated AIDS cases, and an estimated 15–17 percent of sexual partners of hemophiliacs with HIV/AIDS have become infected.

CHAPTER 6

HIV/AIDS AND THE HEALTH-CARE SYSTEM

FINANCING HEALTH-CARE DELIVERY

Care for HIV/AIDS patients is expensive, so even though newer drug treatments—highly active antiretroviral therapy (HAART)—have high per-unit costs, their introduction in 1996 reduced total health care spending on AIDS by reducing the rate of hospitalization and use of outpatient care. According to a study conducted by the Rand Corporation and published in the March 15, 2001 issue of *The New England Journal of Medicine* the average HIV patient incurred costs of about $1,410 per month in 1998. In 1998 a year's worth of drug treatment for HIV could cost as much as $18,000 per patient. Persons with AIDS could spend up to $77,000 per year on medication alone.

Some HIV/AIDS patients rely on health insurance to help pay these costs, but many patients are not insured. Many policies exclude or deny coverage to persons with pre-existing conditions and, as a result, many HIV-positive people are denied private health insurance.

Medicaid (an entitlement program run by the state and federal government to provide health care insurance to patients younger than 65 years who cannot afford to pay for private health insurance) pays the costs of approximately half of all adults and nearly 90 percent of children living with HIV/AIDS, according to the Office of National AIDS Policy, a White House agency. Medicaid eligibility requirements vary from state to state; it generally covers people with incomes of less than $625 per month who cannot engage in substantial gainful employment due to physical or mental impairment that is expected to last at least one year or result in death. Medicaid programs vary widely by jurisdiction; many states supplement federal funding with state funds and each state determines not only the eligibility criteria for its program but also the benefits—the number and type of treatments provided through the program.

A Reverse in Federal Policy

In early 1997 the Clinton administration announced that it hoped to expand Medicaid to cover all low-income HIV-infected people. By the end of the year, however, the administration announced that it could not follow through with this nationwide plan because it would increase government spending. (Both the Clinton administration and subsequent Bush administration forbade the federal government and states to change the Medicaid rules if that change would increase spending over a five-year period.) The administration had hoped to give low-income HIV-positive persons access to HAART drugs that slow the onset of AIDS. Under the present terms of Medicaid, only patients who have been diagnosed with AIDS, not those who are HIV-positive, are covered.

State Programs to Provide Drugs

In the late 1980s state-administered programs were established to help AIDS patients pay for AZT (now called zidovudine or ZDV), the newest effective drug at the time. The programs give free drugs to AIDS patients who are not poor enough to qualify for Medicaid coverage but who do not have private health insurance coverage, or patients who have used up their prescription drug coverage. The federal government provides two-thirds of the funding for the state programs, and the balance comes mostly from the states. In 1996 federal and state drug program expenditures for the fiscal year totaled about $145 million.

Until recently, the programs did not attract many participants, primarily because ZDV alone was not very effective against the disease. In the late 1990s, however, with the development of a new class of antiretroviral drugs—called protease inhibitors (PIs)—that seem to reduce the amount of virus in the blood, more patients wanted to take advantage of the programs. (The typical three-drug cocktail—one new PI combined with two other HIV/AIDS medications—costs at least $12,000 per year per patient.)

This growing demand has put a financial strain on the programs, and many states are having to ration HIV/AIDS drugs or turn patients away in order to remain solvent. Some states are making it harder for people to qualify for the programs, and a few states are beginning to charge small copayments to offset the cost of the drugs. Several states do not offer the new drugs through their programs. More than 30 states offer at least one PI, but 17 states do not provide any. Even after cutbacks in their AIDS drug programs, some states may run out of money before they are expected to receive more federal funds.

Costs to the Insurance Industry

A 1995 survey conducted by the American Council of Life Insurance and the Health Insurance Association of America found that the nation's insurers paid out $1.6 billion in AIDS-related claims during 1994, a 7 percent increase over 1993. Between 1985 and 1994 the insurance companies paid out an estimated $9.4 billion.

INSURANCE CAPS ON HIV/AIDS TREATMENT. Some employers, largely those that are self-insured and paying premiums to third-party insurers as protection against catastrophic health-care claims, have put caps on expenditures for HIV/AIDS treatments. In some cases these employers have reduced their policies from million-dollar lifetime coverage to $10,000, which does not cover a year's worth of treatment. Because self-insured plans are exempt from most states' insurance regulations, employees who acquire HIV have no recourse from insurance caps.

NEW LIFE INSURANCE AVAILABLE. In 1997 the Guarantee Trust Life Insurance Company, a small Midwestern company, began to offer life insurance to some HIV-positive people. Company president Richard S. Holson III said the company decided to offer the coverage because they believe that many HIV-positive people are otherwise healthy and should be viewed as having a treatable chronic illness rather than a terminal disease. With new treatments available, affected people are living longer.

The policies provide up to $250,000 coverage and are offered to those who acquired the virus through sexual activity or accidental needle sticks. Applicants must be between the ages of 21–49, have previous and current CD4 tests of 400 or greater, and never have been diagnosed with AIDS. Coverage is not offered to persons who acquired the disease through the injection of drugs because drug use increases the company's risks, including the chance that prescribed medications will not be taken. The coverage is expensive: a typical 30-year old non-smoking male who is HIV-positive pays $1,500 per month for the $250,000 policy.

Changes to the Health-Care System

Since the 1960s, U.S. government spending on health services has consistently increased. Between 1980 and 1990 federal health expenses rose from 12 percent to 15 percent of the federal budget. At the same time, health-care providers—doctors, hospitals, and other health-related institutions and professions—have watched as payments for Medicare, Medicaid, and private insurance coverage, once easily obtained in the 1960s and 1970s, were increasingly laden with restrictions and limits. Providers also encountered a greater reticence among private insurers to pay in the 1990s. Bureaucratic management, increasing amounts of paperwork to document medical care and claims, and slow reimbursement rates prompted some physicians to stop caring for Medicare/Medicaid patients. Managed-care programs, which often restrict physicians' professional decisions and patient choices, were initially designed to control medical care costs.

Many managed-care programs, also known as health maintenance organizations (HMOs) and preferred provider organizations (PPOs), are having administrative and financial problems. These programs, which rely heavily on primary care practitioners (general and family physicians), are currently re-evaluating the treatment they provide for HIV/AIDS patients. For the first time, large numbers of HIV-infected people are enrolled in managed-care networks, in part because more companies are placing all employees in HMOs and PPOs, and in part because government insurance programs are also directing Medicaid recipients to such programs.

NEW MANAGED-CARE PROGRAM FOR HIV/AIDS PATIENTS—THE TENNESSEE "CENTERS OF EXCELLENCE" PROGRAM. In May 1998 Tennessee Medicaid (TennCare) introduced a voluntary managed-care program for its members with HIV or AIDS. The model program features "Centers of Excellence" providers—practitioners with high levels of expertise in the care of HIV/AIDS patients. The providers must agree to adopt and adhere to a clinical protocol (set of rules) developed by a committee composed of providers, consumers, managed-care organizations, and public health officials. The protocol committee meets up to twice per month to discuss and recommend new drug therapies as they become available and to inform participating providers about new treatments.

Providers may be solo (individual) practitioners with access to needed services or full-service clinics. There are no financial incentives to participate in the program; however, providers who meet the Centers of Excellence criteria do not have to obtain prior authorizations when they prescribe drugs or treatments that fall under the clinical protocols.

The Centers of Excellence program frees managed-care organizations (MCOs) from the clinical and administrative responsibility of keeping close tabs on HIV and AIDS care. It also allows MCOs to remain confident that providers are capable and have access to a wide range of services needed by members. MCO members know that

TABLE 6.1

Office visits, by diagnostic and screening services ordered or provided and patient's sex, 1999

Diagnostic and screening services ordered or provided	Number of visits in thousands[1]	Standard error in thousands	Percent distribution	Standard error of percent	Female[2] Percent distribution	Female Standard error of percent	Male[3] Percent distribution	Male Standard error of percent
All visits	756,734	30,743	...	...	...	...	...	...
None	200,097	13,182	26.4	1.4	24.8	1.5	28.8	1.6
Examinations								
Skin	75,557	6,381	10.0	0.7	9.9	0.8	10.1	1.0
Visual	59,267	5,425	7.8	0.7	7.2	0.7	8.7	0.9
Pelvic	49,720	5,262	6.6	0.6	10.3	1.0	1.2	0.3
Breast	48,835	5,299	6.5	0.6	10.3	1.0	*1.0	0.3
Rectal	30,575	3,163	4.0	0.4	4.0	0.5	4.1	0.4
Glaucoma	29,055	3,857	3.8	0.5	3.7	0.5	4.0	0.5
Hearing	12,395	2,439	1.6	0.3	1.1	0.2	2.4	0.6
Tests								
Blood pressure	339,342	22,079	44.8	1.9	47.2	2.0	41.5	2.0
Urinalysis	62,240	5,388	8.2	0.6	9.0	0.7	7.1	0.8
Hematocrit/hemoglobin	43,452	4,823	5.7	0.6	5.8	0.6	5.7	0.7
Cholesterol	27,035	2,969	3.6	0.4	3.3	0.4	4.0	0.4
Pap test	26,771	2,954	3.5	0.3	6.0	0.6	*	...
EKG[4]	22,593	2,286	3.0	0.3	2.4	0.3	3.8	0.4
Strep test	10,908	2,098	1.4	0.3	1.5	0.3	1.4	0.3
PSA[5]	9,640	947	1.3	0.1	*	...	3.1	0.3
Pregnancy test	3,061	558	0.4	0.1	0.7	0.1	*	...
HIV serology[6]	*2,307	859	*0.3	0.1	*	...	*	...
Blood lead level	*1,631	676	*0.2	0.1	*	...	*	...
Other STD[7]	3,322	962	0.4	0.1	*0.7	0.2	*	...
Other blood test	103,033	7,523	13.6	0.8	14.2	0.8	12.8	0.9
Imaging								
x ray	51,918	3,561	6.9	0.4	6.3	0.4	7.7	0.5
Ultrasound	16,609	2,037	2.2	0.3	2.5	0.4	1.8	0.2
CAT scan/MRI[8,9]	12,778	1,510	1.7	0.2	1.5	0.2	2.0	0.2
Mammography	12,733	1,657	1.7	0.2	2.9	0.3	*	...
Other	102,860	7,718	13.6	1.0	13.4	1.0	13.9	1.1

. . . Category not applicable.
* Figure does not meet standard of reliability or precision.
[1] Number may not add to totals because more than one service may be reported per visit.
[2] Based on 445,566,000 visits made by females.
[3] Based on 311,168,000 visits made by males.
[4] EKG is electrocardiogram.
[5] PSA is prostate-specific antigen.
[6] HIV is human immunodeficiency virus.
[7] STD is sexually transmitted diseases.
[8] CAT is computerized axial tomography.
[9] MRI is magnetic resonance imaging.

SOURCE: Donald K. Cherry, Catharine W. Burt, and David A. Woodwell, "Table 13. Number and percent of office visits with corresponding standard errors, by diagnostic and screening services ordered or provided and patient's sex: United States, 1999," in *National Ambulatory Medical Care Survey: 1999 summary*, National Center for Health Statistics, Hyattsville, MD, 2001

participating providers meet high standards of HIV/AIDS clinical care. Other managed care programs are developing comparable programs to meet the unique health and social service needs of persons living with HIV/AIDS.

Challenges for the Delivery System

HIV/AIDS poses a major challenge to health-care institutions, health-care professionals, and others who provide direct health-care services. HIV/AIDS is a relatively new disease, whereas most medical knowledge is acquired over many years or generations. The health-care system is now caring for about one million persons in the United States suffering from a disease that is still only partly understood. The system must also plan to deliver services to the tens of thousands of people in this country who are HIV-positive today who will require specialized health care services during the coming years, although only a small proportion need intensive medical care at any one time.

The number of indigent people in need of HIV/AIDS care, particularly those who bring the added complications of drug addiction, homelessness, and other socioeconomic problems, has strained public hospitals in particular. Patients in public hospitals are often different from those in private hospitals; they generally seek care later in the course of the disease's progression and are, therefore,

TABLE 6.2

Office visits, by therapeutic and preventive services ordered or provided and patient's sex, 1999

| Therapeutic and preventive services ordered or provided | Number of visits in thousands[1] | Standard error in thousands | Percent of visits | Standard error of percent | Patient's sex | | | |
| | | | | | Female[2] | | Male[3] | |
					Percent of visits	Standard error of percent	Percent of visits	Standard error of percent
All visits	756,734	30,743	...	...	...	...	...	...
None	513,788	23,494	67.9	1.3	66.6	1.5	69.7	1.4
Counseling/education								
Diet	103,885	9,417	13.7	1.0	14.4	1.2	12.8	1.0
Exercise	74,005	6,911	9.8	0.8	10.0	0.9	9.4	0.8
Injury prevention	22,842	4,442	3.0	0.6	2.5	0.5	3.8	1.0
Tobacco use/exposure	21,717	3,019	2.9	0.4	2.6	0.3	3.3	0.5
Stress management	17,320	2,914	2.3	0.4	2.3	0.3	2.3	0.5
Mental health	16,631	2,507	2.2	0.3	2.2	0.3	2.2	0.4
Growth/development	16,034	2,669	2.1	0.3	1.9	0.4	2.4	0.4
Skin cancer prevention	14,611	2,656	1.9	0.3	1.9	0.4	1.9	0.4
Breast self-examination	10,089	1,342	1.3	0.2	2.2	0.3	*	...
Family planning/contraception	8,428	1,216	1.1	0.2	1.7	0.2	*	...
Prenatal instructions	8,399	1,753	1.1	0.2	1.9	0.4	*	...
HIV/STD transmission[4,5]	5,034	860	0.7	0.1	0.7	0.1	0.6	0.2
Other therapy								
Psycho-pharmacotherapy	26,343	3,129	3.5	0.4	3.4	0.4	3.6	0.4
Psychotherapy	20,711	3,104	2.7	0.4	2.8	0.4	2.7	0.4
Physiotherapy	18,279	2,706	2.4	0.3	2.4	0.4	2.4	0.4
Alternative medicine	2,922	783	0.4	0.1	0.4	0.1	*0.3	0.1
Other	24,878	2,690	3.3	0.4	3.1	0.4	3.5	0.3

. . . Category not applicable.
* Figure does not meet standard of reliability or precision.
[1] Numbers may not add to totals because more than one type of therapeutic or preventative service may be reported per visit.
[2] Based on 445,556,000 visits made by females.
[3] Based on 311,168,000 visits made by males.
[4] HIV is human immunodeficiency virus.
[5] STD is sexually transmitted disease.

SOURCE: Donald K. Cherry, Catharine W. Burt, and David A. Woodwell, "Table 14. Number and percent of office visits with corresponding standard errors, by therapeutic and preventive services ordered or provided and patient's sex: United States, 1999," in *National Ambulatory Medical Care Survey: 1999 summary,* National Center for Health Statistics, Hyattsville, MD, 2001

sicker. The scarcity of resources—trained personnel, hospital beds, and support services—in the community, combined with inadequate funding and reimbursement for HIV/AIDS care, are significant obstacles to effective health care delivery for indigent HIV/AIDS patients.

OFFICE VISITS. Some physicians, particularly those with many HIV/AIDS patients, have extended their office hours or hired counselors to deal with these patients because their visits are time-consuming. In 1999 physicians polled by the Centers for Disease Control and Prevention (CDC) (Donald K. Cherry, Catharine W. Burt, and David A. Woodwell, "National Ambulatory Medical Care Survey: 1999 Summary," *Advance Data,* No. 322, July 17, 2001) reported more than 2 million patient visits for HIV in 1999. (See Table 6.1.) While this represented less than 0.2 percent of the estimated 757 million visits for all causes in 1999, it did not reflect the growing amount of time spent on diagnostic and screening services in each office, or the increase in the number of visits devoted to counseling and educating HIV/AIDS patients. According to the same survey, 5.7 million office visits provided counseling for and education about HIV and STD transmission (0.7 percent of all patient visits). (See Table 6.2.)

HOSPITAL CARE. The nation's 7,000 hospitals are also feeling the pinch of Medicare rate limits, reduced payments from MCOs, and intense competition from other providers, such as ambulatory surgical centers and hospices; and many are struggling to remain profitable institutions. During the 1970s and 1980s the steady growth of "for-profit" hospitals lured many privately insured, middle-class patients away from community hospitals, leaving most of the uninsured, sicker patients to seek care from inner-city public hospitals.

Most HIV/AIDS patients are cared for in inner-city public hospitals that are already overburdened with inadequate revenues, staff shortages, lack of referral facilities, and emergency rooms used by many poor neighborhood residents as sources of primary medical care. Many health-care professionals praise San Francisco's model of care. The California city was hit hard in the early days of the epidemic and developed a range of innovative, effective programs in response to acute need during the early 1990s. This model of care relies on extensive out-patient services and volunteer social support services provided by the well-established and well-organized gay and lesbian community.

CHANGES IN HEALTH-CARE DELIVERY. Although fewer persons are acquiring HIV/AIDS, the evolution of HIV care is altering the ways in which health care is delivered. In the late stages of AIDS, most patients require intermittent hospitalization and home health care. Those who are not as severely affected and have symptoms or conditions that once required intravenous therapy (which had to be administered in a hospital or by home health professionals) are now able to self-medicate at home. Many drugs are now available for oral administration in pill or liquid form. All these home care and community-based measures lessen the burden on the health care delivery system and make it easier for HIV/AIDS patients to care for themselves.

Persons with AIDS (PWAs) who receive informal home health care (care from friends and family) often use fewer hospital services; and this may reflect a greater desire to remain at home. PWAs with strong social support systems and who prefer to remain at home may also be less likely to demand an aggressive approach to treating their illness. Those who receive formal home health care (visits from physicians, nurses, therapists, social workers, case managers, and other paid caregivers) often use more hospital services. This may reflect a greater use of all types of health services by PWAs with weaker social support systems and/or an aggressive approach to treatment by medical professionals.

AN AIDS CARE ALTERNATIVE. In 1993, in an effort to offer Atlanta's 4,400 uninsured AIDS patients treatment equal to that available to patients with private insurance, Grady Memorial Hospital opened a $7 million outpatient HIV/AIDS clinic. The clinic and its 150-member staff provide emergency care, dental services, mental health counseling, social and support services, HIV research and education, case management, and babysitting. The clinic is partially financed under a provision of the Ryan White CARE Act of 1990 (PL 101-381), enacted to provide funding to improve the quality and availability of care for HIV-infected people. In 1994 the clinic began asking patients to pay nominal fees based on their incomes. Under the CARE act, providers may charge up to 10 percent of a patient's wages.

HOSPICE CARE. The AIDS epidemic has had a significant impact on hospices. Hospice care, both in the home and in specialized centers, offers palliative care aimed at comfort rather than cure. This includes expert pain relief, along with emotional, psychological, and spiritual support for patients, their families, and friends. The majority of hospice patients are older adults, suffer from terminal diseases such as cancer, and face imminent death.

Historically, AIDS patients did not fit well into hospices. AIDS patients were younger than traditional hospice patients; and their disease progresses less predictably than many cancers. Further, as one hospice administrator noted, because many people with AIDS were accustomed to prejudice, they initially mistrusted the motivation and altruism of hospice workers. Today, more than two decades after the first cases of AIDS were identified, home-based hospice programs designed to meet the needs of AIDS patients, their partners, and families have gained acceptance in the medical community as well as among HIV-infected persons and the voluntary social service agencies organized to support them.

HEALTH-CARE PROVIDERS

Physicians

The Social Impact of AIDS in the United States (Albert J. Jonsen and Jedd Stryker, eds., National Academy Press, Washington, D.C., 1993) described "AIDS physicians" as doctors who perform a wide variety of services in addition to providing care to AIDS patients. Many are also AIDS activists and may be involved in developing policies, planning for care needs, and dealing with the media.

One challenge of training physicians to treat AIDS patients is that AIDS care requires skills and training in the multitude of conditions known to be part of HIV/AIDS disease. However, the amount of experience—rather than the kind of training—may be a better predictor of the quality of care the physician is able to deliver.

A study presented at the Third Annual Conference on Retroviruses and Opportunistic Infections in Washington, D.C., was cited in "Survival of Patients with AIDS Depends on Physicians' Experience Treating the Disease" (*The Journal of the American Medical Association,* Vol. 275, No. 10, March 13, 1996). The study claimed that AIDS patients treated by primary care physicians with no previous experience treating AIDS patients died more than a year earlier than those whose doctors had treated at least five AIDS patients. The study also showed patients had a 46 percent decrease in relative risk of death at any given time when treated by a physician who had treated other AIDS patients. The difference, according to the researchers, was that the more experienced physicians consulted more frequently with physician specialists and reported more visits with their AIDS patients.

FEWER PHYSICIANS RELUCTANT TO TREAT HIV PATIENTS. Unfortunately, the AIDS epidemic began at a time when many newly graduated physicians were not choosing primary care specialties such as internal medicine, the most fitting for the ongoing care required by

HIV-infected patients. Some observers feared that new physicians would avoid practicing in geographic areas where there are large proportions of HIV/AIDS patients.

Fortunately, the CDC has found that most primary care doctors believe that they have an obligation to care for HIV-infected patients and are interested in further professional training to help increase their skill and comfort in caring for HIV/AIDS patients. Among physicians who report they do not provide care to AIDS patients, the majority cite a lack of experience with HIV and note that providers with more expertise are readily available in their communities.

Nurses

Social Impact observed that it is more difficult to assess the impact of HIV/AIDS on nurses than on doctors. It appears that nurses often have different viewpoints than some physicians about their professional obligations to patients with HIV. As hospital employees, nurses seldom have the option of choosing whether to treat a particular patient (nor do patients have much choice of nurses). Nurses, however, report that caring for HIV/AIDS patients can take an enormous emotional toll since they are often the primary source of continuous physical and emotional care of persons with HIV/AIDS, who generally require more care and services than other patients.

Nurses, physicians, and other health care professionals must cope with more than simply their fears of contracting the disease from HIV/AIDS patients and keeping abreast of advances in the treatment of HIV disease. They also face a wide range of emotional issues when caring for these patients, from feelings of "failure" when treatment is unsuccessful to grief when witnessing the untimely deaths of patients. Support groups and counselors help many health professionals, especially hospice workers, to share and understand these feelings so they are better able to care for HIV/AIDS patients and their families.

CDC Guidelines

In 1992, in response to an incident in which five patients acquired HIV from a Florida dentist, the CDC addressed occupational exposure to blood-borne pathogens. The CDC offered new guidelines to prevent the accidental spread of the infection from health-care providers to patients and from patients to health-care workers. The recommendations stressed the careful and consistent use, with all patients, of standard infection control procedures for blood-borne agents—the so-called "universal precautions."

The guidelines also recommended that HIV-infected health-care workers cease performing what were termed "exposure-prone invasive procedures" and that professional medical and dental groups draw up lists of "exposure-prone procedures" for their disciplines. The CDC recommended that HIV-infected health-care workers consult with a panel of experts to determine which, if any, limits should be placed on their medical practices and further advised practitioners to inform patients of their HIV-infection status before performing medical procedures.

The CDC guidelines resulted in some unforeseen consequences. Professional groups, hospital attorneys, state courts, legislatures, and the U.S. Congress reacted with alarm to a perception of dangers to patients posed by HIV-infected health-care professionals totally out of proportion to the largely theoretical risk. According to the U.S. Public Health Service, the average risk of HIV infection after skin contact with HIV-infected blood is estimated to be about 0.3 percent; and the risk for transmission is probably even lower from contact with body fluids or tissues other than blood. Through 1990, 40 cases of occupationally acquired HIV were documented; by June 2000, 56 documented cases had been reported, and 138 additional cases of HIV infection are considered possibly linked to occupational exposures.

Most medical professional associations refused to cooperate in developing a list of exposure-prone invasive procedures that carry a higher risk of virus transmission. They did not believe there was enough data to support drawing up such a list. Nonetheless, the CDC did not withdraw its recommendation concerning the exposure-prone procedures list, even after studies of more than 15,000 patients taken care of by 32 health-care workers known to be HIV-infected found that none of the patients contracted HIV as a result of the care.

The CDC also recommended that the following procedures and philosophies would best serve patients and health-care workers:

- The universal and meticulous use of well-understood infection control procedures, particularly those developed from the study of hepatitis B—another blood-borne infection that is one hundred times more infectious and 10 times more common in health professionals—should be applied in all health-care settings, whether hospital, office, or home-based.

- Operative or other invasive procedures in which injury to health-care professionals occurs with any frequency should be discontinued or modified to the extent possible. This involves developing new instruments and investigating new operative techniques.

- All health-care professionals should consider being tested for HIV. An HIV-positive result, however, should not justify restricting the practice of health-care professionals.

The National Commission on AIDS did not agree with all of the CDC guidelines, cautioning against placing too much emphasis on HIV transmission in health-care settings. Unwarranted emphasis in the wrong place, noted the Commission, distracts the nation from proper attention to sexual transmission, transmission via injection drug use, the problems of sexually active teenagers, and an epidemic that needs more committed health-care professionals.

The Commission also warned that the costs associated with testing all health-care professionals and all patients would amount to $1.5 billion and that there was no evidence that such testing would increase patient or worker safety. In *Preventing HIV Transmission in Healthcare Settings* (Washington, D.C., 1992), the Commission further stated,

> The determination that an HIV-infected health-care worker is not able to continue to practice medicine or otherwise work with patients should be based on an individualized review. Criteria for action should include whether or not the worker is able to comply with universal precautions and infection control guidelines and procedures, lacks professional competence and/or judgment, or has been responsible for documented transmission of other blood-borne infections.

> The Commission is acutely aware of the magnitude and intensity of public alarm. Indeed, public polls have indicated that over 90 percent of Americans believe their doctors should tell them if they, the physicians, are HIV-positive. Those polled further indicate that they would not make use of the services of an HIV-infected doctor. This is a reality we must face. It shows how poorly we have informed our citizenry.

> The Commission believes it is important to acknowledge forthrightly fears concerning HIV transmission in the health-care setting and address them, without allowing them to overwhelm rational judgment. Policies must be directed at eliminating risks that are significant rather than remote or theoretical. Policies must be grounded in scientific reality and be sufficiently flexible to respond to new scientific evidence. To this end, the Commission offers a set of guiding principles that will endure should new evidence come to light. The promotion of patient safety and access to health care must remain paramount concerns. The "cure" for the risk of HIV transmission in the health-care setting must not be more damaging than the risk itself to the public's health.

Should Doctors Tell Patients?

Since 1991, the American College of Surgeons (ACS), the nation's largest professional organization of surgeons, in defiance of the CDC guidelines, has refused to draw up a list of procedures that might pose a high risk of transmitting HIV from doctor to patient. The group maintains that since not a single documented case of surgeon-to-patient transmission has been established, there is no scientific basis for suggesting that a particular surgical procedure increases the risk of viral transmission. The ACS also noted that surgical patients are at greater risk for other surgery-related infections than for HIV, even from an HIV-infected physician.

HEALTH-CARE WORKERS AND INFECTION

Health-Care Workers with HIV and AIDS

By June 2000 the CDC was aware of only 56 documented cases of health-care workers in the United States who had become infected with HIV as a result of occupational exposures. The CDC is also aware of between 130 and 140 cases of HIV infection or AIDS among health-care workers. These workers have not reported other risk factors for HIV infection. They have reported a history of occupational exposure to blood, body fluids, or HIV-infected laboratory material, but have not documented infection after a specific exposure. Although the CDC is aware of between 130 and 140 cases, there are undoubtedly unknown others who acquired their infection through occupational exposures.

As of October 2000, 15 states had enacted needle-safety legislation to safeguard health care workers from bloodborne pathogen (agents that cause disease) exposures. State laws aim to strengthen and supplement the federal standards mandated by the Occupational Safety and Health Administration (OSHA). Many of the state laws require the creation of: a written exposure plan that is periodically reviewed and updated; protocols for safety device identification and selection; logs to document and report injuries with sharp instruments; and strict requirements and training for workers on how to use safety devices.

In 2001, the U.S. Public Health Service updated guidelines for treatment to prevent health care workers with occupational exposure to HIV from becoming infected with the virus. Known as "postexposure prophylaxis" (PEP), the recommendation is that affected workers be given a four-week regimen of two antiretroviral drugs such as zidovudine and lamivudine, with the addition of a third drug for HIV exposures that pose an increased risk of transmission. While the best strategy to protect health care workers from HIV is to avoid exposure to HIV and other bloodborne pathogens, PEP has, to date, proven effective in preventing HIV infection in workers who have been exposed.

Risks to Patients

Health-care officials are not the only ones worried about HIV transmission in the health-care setting. Patients also fear that infected health-care workers could transmit the virus to them. The CDC has developed a model of the risk of HIV transmission to patients and estimated that the risk of a patient's becoming infected by an HIV-infected surgeon during a single operation is between 1 in 42,000 and 1 in 420,000. This risk is considerably less than the risks associated with many other medical procedures.

Ongoing studies by the CDC of more than 15,700 patients of 32 HIV-infected health-care workers have found *no* documented evidence that HIV infections found in these studies could be attributed to medical or dental care, with the exception of the five patients of a Florida dentist in 1990. Medical researchers have tried without success to determine how the dentist infected his patients and whether the exposure was accidental or deliberate. One theory is that he did not properly sterilize his dental tools; another is that he accidentally cut his finger or jabbed himself with a hypodermic needle, did not notice it and bled into the patients' mouths. Prior to his death in 1990, the dentist denied intentionally exposing his patients.

In 1990, Dr. Rudolph Almarez, a Baltimore breast surgeon who performed operations on as many as 2,000 patients, died from AIDS. His situation stirred up such concern that shortly after his death, a Baltimore law firm solicited clients to seek legal advice, whether they were infected or not. The law firm told clients that they might be reimbursed for the emotional distress they now suffered if they sued the hospital where Dr. Almarez had practiced. A Baltimore judge, in two separate cases, dismissed complaints based on the fear of HIV exposure. The judge further stated that there were no allegations that Dr. Almarez had not followed recommended safety procedures or that any accident had taken place during surgery. None of the patients alleged infection from Dr. Almarez. A later study failed to find any HIV-positive patients among those Dr. Almarez had treated. (*Rossi v. Almarez*, *Faya v. Almarez*, Baltimore City Cir. Ct. Nos. 90344028 CL123396; 90345011 CL12345g, May 23, 1991).

CHAPTER 7
COST, TREATMENT, AND RESEARCH

WHAT DOES IT COST TO TREAT HIV/AIDS PATIENTS?

The treatment of HIV/AIDS is expensive. Barney Graham, a scientific investigator at Vanderbilt University in Tennessee, estimates that HIV/AIDS costs the United States approximately $13 million each day. In 1996 the AIDS research budget for the National Institute for Allergy and Infectious Diseases (NIAID) was $1.4 billion. A full-scale clinical trial for a new drug costs between $9 million and $18 million. The per-patient cost of HIV/AIDS drugs is between $12,000 and $70,000 a year depending on the severity of the patient's condition; costs are expected to increase due to the rising costs of hospitalization, home care, insurance premiums and copayments, and physician services. Additionally, federal and state programs such as Medicaid have been forced to operate under tighter budgets and have eliminated certain treatments from insurance coverage. During 2000 certain drugs (including Bristol-Myers Squibb's new enteric coated formulation of didanosine, or ddI, and Abbott Labs' new protease inhibitor ABT-378) rose substantially in price.

Some expenses, however, have actually been reduced by relocating services from the hospital to a variety of outpatient settings. Examples of cost-saving services include outpatient transfusions and outpatient treatment for opportunistic infections such as *Pneumocystis carinii* pneumonia (PCP) and cryptococcal meningitis. Increased volunteer-based social service programs that enable patients to be cared for at home also serve to prevent expensive hospital stays.

Federal government spending on HIV-related care and activities has increased steadily since 1985, when about $2 million was spent. In 2000 the Budget Office of the Public Health Service estimated that federal spending for HIV-related expenses was nearly $11 billion, $6.3 billion of which was spent on medical care. Other government costs included research ($2.1 billion), education and prevention ($1 billion), and cash assistance ($1.4 billion), which is provided through the Social Security Administration and the Department of Housing and Urban Development. (See Table 7.1.)

The Ryan White Comprehensive AIDS Resources Emergency (CARE) Act

In 1998 the Ryan White CARE Act (PL 101-381) was the only federal program providing funds specifically for medical and support services to individuals with HIV and AIDS. (Ryan White, who died of AIDS in 1990, was an Indiana teenager who received national attention because he was shunned by many people in his community who feared he would infect their children.) The Act was signed in 1990 and reauthorized in 1996 and 2000. The 2000 reauthorization addressed additional initiatives including: improving access to care for vulnerable populations (such as women, minorities, and those with addictions or mental health disorders); increased accountability of providers; and improving services in underserved rural and urban regions.

CARE funds are appropriated using four formulas. The Title I formula provides emergency assistance to metropolitan areas disproportionately affected by the HIV epidemic. To qualify for Title I funds, eligible metropolitan areas (EMAs) must have more than 2,000 cumulative AIDS cases reported during the preceding five years and a population of at least 500,000. (The population provision does not apply to any EMA named and funded before fiscal year [FY] 1997.) In FY 1991, the first year Title I grants were available, there were only 19 EMAs; in FY 2001 there were 51 EMAs in 22 states, the District of Columbia, and Puerto Rico. Since its inception in FY 1991, more than $3.6 billion in Title I funding has been allotted; in FY 2001 EMAs received $582.7 million. New York ($119.3 million), San Francisco ($35.7 million), and Los Angeles ($35 million) received the largest grants. (see Table 7.2.)

TABLE 7.1

Federal spending for HIV-related activities, according to agency and type of activity, selected fiscal years 1985–2000

[Data are compiled from Federal Government appropriations]

Agency and type of activity	1985	1990	1995	1996	1997	1998	1999	2000[1]
Agency				Amount in millions				
All Federal spending	$205	$3,064	$6,821	$7,522	$8,363	$8,931	$9,966	$10,932
Department of Health and Human Services, total	197	2,620	4,941	5,598	6,367	6,835	7,694	8,488
Department of Health and Human Services discretionary spending, total[2]	109	1,591	2,700	2,898	3,267	3,535	4,094	4,588
National Institutes of Health	66	907	1,334	1,411	1,501	1,604	1,793	2,006
Substance Abuse and Mental Health Services Administration	–	50	24	54	64	70	92	114
Centers for Disease Control and Prevention	33	443	590	584	617	625	657	730
Food and Drug Administration	9	57	73	73	73	73	70	70
Health Resources and Services Administration	–	113	661	762	1,001	1,155	1,416	1,600
Agency for Health Care Policy and Research	–	8	9	6	4	1	2	3
Office of Public Health and Science[3]	–	8	4	4	4	4	12	12
Indian Health Service	–	3	4	3	4	4	4	4
Emergency Fund	...	...	...	...	...	...	50	50
Other Department of Health and Human Services agencies	–	3	2	2	–	–	–	–
Health Care Financing Administration	75	780	2,240	2,700	3,100	3,300	3,600	3,900
Social Security Administration[4]	13	249	...	...	...	...	...	...
Social Security Administration[4]	...	...	940	976	1,001	1,061	1,149	1,177
Department of Veterans Affairs	8	220	317	331	332	343	401	457
Department of Defense	–	125	112	98	100	105	86	98
Agency for International Development	–	71	120	115	117	121	135	190
Department of Housing and Urban Development	–	–	171	171	196	204	225	232
Office of Personnel Management	–	21	212	226	241	253	266	279
Other departments	–	7	8	7	9	9	10	11
Activity								
Research	84	1,142	1,589	1,653	1,730	1,831	1,900	2,124
Department of Health and Human Services discretionary spending[2]	83	1,093	1,544	1,619	1,702	1,801	1,869	2,083
Department of Veterans Affairs	1	15	5	6	6	6	7	7
Department of Defense	–	34	40	28	22	24	24	34
Education and prevention	26	486	658	635	685	701	918	1,057
Department of Health and Human Services discretionary spending[2]	25	351	492	476	522	534	739	820
Department of Veterans Affairs	1	31	31	31	31	31	30	33
Department of Defense	–	28	12	11	12	13	10	10
Agency for International Development	–	71	120	115	117	121	135	190
Other	–	5	3	2	3	2	4	4
Medical care	81	1,187	3,462	4,087	4,752	5,134	5,775	6,342
Health Care Financing Administration:								
Medicaid (Federal share)	70	670	1,640	1,600	1,800	1,900	2,100	2,200
Medicare	5	110	600	1,100	1,300	1,400	1,500	1,700
Department of Health and Human Services discretionary spending[2]	–	144	664	803	1,044	1,200	1,487	1,685
Department of Veterans Affairs	6	174	281	294	295	306	364	417
Department of Defense	–	63	60	59	66	68	52	54
Office of Personnel Management "	–	21	212	226	241	253	266	279
Other	–	5	5	5	6	7	6	7
Cash assistance	13	249	1,111	1,147	1,197	1,265	1,374	1,409
Social Security Administration:								
Disability Insurance	10	210	640	696	691	726	789	792
Supplemental Security Income	3	39	300	280	310	335	360	385
Department of Housing and Urban Development	–	–	171	171	196	204	225	232

– Quantity zero.
... Category not applicable.
[1] Preliminary figures.
[2] Department of Health and Human Services discretionary spending is spending that is not entitlement spending. Medicare and Medicaid are examples of entitlement spending.
[3] The Office of the Assistant Secretary for Health prior to FY 1996.
[4] Prior to 1995 the Social Security Administration was part of the Department of Health and Human Services.

SOURCE: "Table 127. Federal spending for human immunodeficiency virus (HIV)-related activities, according to agency and type of activity: United States, selected fiscal years 1985–2000," in *Health, United States, 2001*, National Center for Health Statistics, Hyattsville, MD, 2001

TABLE 7.2

Ryan White CARE Act Title I grant awards, 1993–2001

Eligible metropolitan area	FY 1993	FY 1994	FY 1995	FY 1996	FY 1997	FY 1998	FY 1999	FY 2000	FY 2001
Atlanta GA	$5,490,571	$7,488,801	$9,091,331	$9,208,162	$12,632,117	$12,021,454	$13,147,268	$15,507,832	$15,992,692
Austin TX	N/E [1]	N/E	2,124,274	2,398,671	3,337,861	2,856,752	3,175,509	3,575,995	3,922,582
Baltimore MD	3,250,343	3,923,438	4,715,150	8,364,074	10,033,688	12,184,481	13,478,549	15,351,112	16,698,367
Bergen-Passaic NJ	N/E	2,019,121	2,847,639	3,369,095	4,292,593	4,354,291	4,320,176	4,626,995	5,234,104
Boston MA	4,154,744	6,955,035	7,079,242	8,360,436	9,033,443	9,463,130	10,647,381	12,469,255	15,363,160
Caguas PR	N/E	N/E	902,928	1,064,876	1,431,210	1,405,197	1,610,314	1,713,686	1,750,404
Chicago IL	7,390,763	9,625,451	12,099,865	13,164,930	15,741,071	15,995,512	18,227,884	19,003,954	22,963,079
Cleveland-Lorain-Elyria OH	N/E	N/E	N/E	1,384,956	1,877,513	2,459,443	2,933,058	3,107,796	3,384,855
Dallas TX	4,542,034	6,935,644	8,176,385	7,820,653	8,129,583	9,082,217	10,164,078	11,077,000	12,098,406
Denver CO	N/E	3,375,884	3,092,041	3,549,707	4,668,572	4,278,161	4,150,341	4,581,734	4,840,128
Detroit MI	2,091,739	2,849,559	2,406,902	4,405,380	6,087,121	5,628,350	6,585,744	7,234,813	7,612,631
Dutchess Co. NY	N/E	N/E	609,583	581,761	776,847	854,481	1,220,662	1,208,858	1,362,331
Ft. Lauderdale FL	4,591,215	6,814,599	5,091,994	6,584,204	8,312,185	10,128,631	10,810,324	11,437,539	13,816,037
Ft. Worth-Arlington TX	N/E	N/E	N/E	2,255,398	1,902,232	2,618,024	2,935,543	2,968,606	3,298,024
Hartford CT	N/E	N/E	N/E	3,048,467	2,661,473	3,613,029	4,019,409	4,417,574	4,868,180
Houston TX	7,820,319	10,133,592	10,233,981	10,312,524	10,768,697	12,722,479	15,489,996	17,665,434	19,283,756
Jacksonville FL	N/E	N/E	2,418,868	2,725,251	3,762,713	3,443,168	3,683,146	4,175,873	4,799,813
Jersey City NJ	3,618,220	4,140,141	3,770,366	3,767,874	4,600,103	5,320,300	5,015,785	5,541,714	6,167,889
Kansas City MO	N/E	2,655,564	2,726,195	2,514,291	2,884,537	2,622,409	2,952,910	3,064,120	3,386,127
Las Vegas NV [2]	0	0	0	0	0	0	3,402,697	3,689,337	4,455,787
Los Angeles CA	19,190,269	25,441,211	31,037,580	26,313,561	30,227,298	30,637,106	33,540,737	34,683,327	35,020,216
Miami FL	9,716,264	15,258,563	19,195,347	15,156,078	18,863,208	18,472,153	21,248,387	23,450,383	25,385,904
Middlesex -Somerset -Hunterdon NJ	N/E	N/E	N/E	2,198,883	1,919,076	2,597,923	2,555,029	2,750,975	2,888,808
Minneapolis-St. Paul MN	N/E	N/E	N/E	1,370,726	1,990,700	2,570,712	2,548,603	2,826,949	3,216,026
Nassau-Suffolk NY	2,012,809	2,886,968	3,895,849	3,683,885	4,697,795	4,939,871	5,632,012	6,118,736	6,532,144
Newark NJ	3,542,848	7,009,180	11,791,405	9,725,848	11,612,530	12,630,257	14,390,269	14,554,092	16,254,538
New Haven CT	N/E	2,136,872	2,711,634	4,002,182	5,336,678	5,348,730	6,100,471	6,261,941	6,944,353
New Orleans LA	1,796,972	3,243,332	3,503,009	2,087,199	4,727,682	4,921,857	5,695,360	5,935,834	6,942,652
New York NY	44,469,219	100,054,267	93,587,184	92,241,697	92,459,373	95,325,334	96,961,856	107,560,148	119,256,891
Norfolk VA [2]	0	0	0	0	0	0	3,665,087	4,089,698	4,736,759
Oakland CA	2,602,816	3,929,287	4,148,299	4,741,595	5,905,961	5,926,194	6,218,532	6,704,657	6,776,406
Orange County CA	1,839,726	2,627,947	3,175,288	3,492,993	4,401,330	3,810,759	4,300,690	4,670,880	4,956,671
Orlando FL	N/E	2,715,587	3,194,835	3,599,489	4,319,349	4,609,839	4,907,180	6,007,600	6,497,014
Philadelphia PA	4,729,230	7,374,936	9,836,096	10,345,478	13,465,328	14,081,773	16,011,451	18,134,011	22,114,655
Phoenix AZ	N/E	2,217,471	2,447,784	2,901,602	3,380,053	3,412,037	3,865,319	5,001,568	6,575,645
Ponce PR	1,280,364	1,176,793	1,908,071	1,685,036	2,183,463	2,200,114	2,487,768	2,460,695	2,607,961
Portland OR	N/E	N/E	2,402,734	2,688,924	3,472,480	3,057,466	3,115,251	3,216,312	3,513,044
Riverside-San Bernardino CA	N/E	2,402,010	2,656,331	4,687,432	5,986,979	5,634,427	6,463,388	6,913,948	6,940,381
Sacramento CA	N/E	N/E	N/E	2,463,814	2,038,827	2,389,370	2,578,873	2,744,171	2,899,765
St. Louis MO	N/E	2,248,247	2,581,330	2,587,364	3,506,350	3,561,850	3,664,771	4,239,080	4,432,316
San Antonio TX	N/E	N/E	1,731,222	2,396,426	3,014,191	2,952,239	3,014,654	3,163,374	3,862,398
San Diego CA	3,761,979	5,233,574	5,628,252	6,592,104	8,198,109	8,452,437	8,872,685	9,071,625	10,577,352
an Francisco CA	18,944,229	27,217,076	39,210,400	35,172,274	37,194,634	36,394,914	36,218,513	35,246,477	35,771,651
San Jose CA	N/E	N/E	N/E	2,275,044	1,992,602	2,445,480	2,486,136	2,612,060	2,866,655
San Juan PR	4,679,777	8,456,057	10,269,416	8,199,506	10,550,845	11,658,912	11,912,865	13,558,330	15,094,482
Santa Rosa-Petaluma CA	N/E	N/E	1,207,605	1,142,456	1,330,630	1,225,807	1,127,018	1,152,406	1,206,194
Seattle WA	2,824,570	3,233,903	4,048,484	4,289,545	5,481,431	5,060,533	5,303,343	5,488,688	5,852,286
Tampa-St. Petersburg FL	2,265,553	3,304,312	4,231,119	4,610,201	6,548,952	6,536,189	7,236,728	8,016,131	8,595,830
Vineland-Millville-Bridgeton NJ	N/E	N/E	340,644	454,338	677,001	594,001	688,648	684,897	807,157
Washington DC	7,447,578	9,328,712	10,713,183	12,763,696	15,838,868	16,710,726	18,322,558	19,903,750	24,507,346
West Palm Beach FL	N/E	3,582,542	3,770,641	3,390,914	5,122,618	5,965,481	6,711,944	7,169,030	7,795,848
TOTALS	**$182,326,998**	**$319,989,000**	**$349,370,000**	**$372,141,000**	**$429,377,900**	**$445,176,000**	**$485,816,900**	**$526,811,000**	**$582,727,700**

[1] "N/E" means the eligible metropolitan area was "not eligible" to receive funding in that fiscal year.
[2] Fiscal year 1999 was the first year of Title I funding.
Note: FY 1991 total was $86,083,000; FY 1992 $119,426,000.

SOURCE: "Ryan White CARE Act Title I Grant Awards," in *Ryan White CARE Act Funding History,* Health Resources and Services Administration, Rockville, MD, January 2001 [Online] ftp://ftp.hrsa.gov/hab/fundinghistory.pdf [accessed December, 2001]

Title II funds are provided to state governments. Ninety percent of Title II funds are distributed on the basis of AIDS patient counts, while 10 percent are distributed through competitive grants awarded to public and nonprofit agencies. More than $4 billion in Title II funding has been allotted since FY 1991. (States that have more than 1 percent of all AIDS cases reported nationally during the preceding two years must match the federal grant with their own resources. The amount is based on an annual formula.) The states use their Title II funds to contract with service providers for ambulatory (outpatient) health care, insurance coverage, residential and in-home hospice care, transportation to and from care appointments, food banks, and home delivered meals. Table 7.3 shows Title II grant funding through FY 2001.

In addition to the base award granted under Title II, states receive funds to support AIDS Drug Assistance Programs (ADAPs). ADAPs provide medication to low-income persons with HIV disease who are either uninsured or underinsured. (The states may elect to use their Title II funds for ADAP.) Beginning in 1996 extra funds were made available for the ADAPs. In FY 1999 a total of $709.9 million (including $461 million for ADAP funding) was allocated for improved health care and support services for people living with HIV/AIDS. Additionally, 1999 was the first year that Guam and the Virgin Islands received ADAP funding. For FY 2001 the amount earmarked for ADAP was $589 million. FY 2001 also was the first year when 3 percent of the ADAP allocation was directed to fund supplemental drug grants to states demonstrating severe need.

Title III of the CARE Act funds grants to provide early intervention services and outpatient treatment for low-income, medically underserved people and supports development of quality HIV primary care programs. During 1999, Title III grants served 108,945 patients; more than two-thirds were people of color. Title IV funds link primary health care and social services for women, infants, and children to HIV research and clinical drug trials. For FY 2001, $185.9 million was allocated to Title III programs and $65 million was appropriated for Title IV programs.

Private Insurance and Medicaid

The financing of HIV/AIDS care is increasingly becoming the responsibility of Medicaid, a government program designed to provide medical care for persons who demonstrate means-tested need. Increasing reliance on Medicaid funding is due in large part to the increase in the number of HIV/AIDS cases among intravenous drug users (IDUs) and poor people who are least likely to be covered by private health insurance. In addition many patients who once had private insurance through their workplace lost their coverage when the illness made them too sick to work, forcing them to turn to Medicaid and other public programs.

Added to this list are those whose employment or economic status would normally assure them insurance coverage, but once they tested positive for HIV they became virtually ineligible for private health insurance coverage. Others need assistance because some insurance companies declare HIV infection a "pre-existing condition," making it ineligible for payment of claims. Even insurance companies that do cover HIV treatment often impose caps, limiting coverage to relatively small dollar amounts.

The HIV/AIDS epidemic has prompted private insurers to add an HIV antibody screening test for people who are not joining insurance programs via groups or employers. These "individual enrollees"—who make up 15 percent of all individuals in the insurance market— are required to take medical exams to prove they are "insur-able." During the early 1990s California, Massachusetts, and the District of Columbia banned the use of HIV antibody testing for private insurance purposes, but the resulting controversy forced them to reverse the ban.

Death Benefits

Since 1988 an industry has developed which offers dying AIDS patients the opportunity to collect a portion of their life insurance benefits before they die, either to pay for their treatment or to spend as they wish during their remaining time. These viatical (money for necessities given to a person dying or in danger of death) settlements are reached when an insured person sells his or her life insurance policy to an independent insurance company at a reduced or discounted price. This enables the patient to have some cash from the policy while he or she is still alive. After the patient dies the company that bought the policy is paid the full death benefits. Regulators with the Securities and Exchange Commission are scrutinizing some practices that they say may victimize AIDS patients.

Some larger companies such as Prudential offer policyholders more than 90 percent of their policy payouts, but only with a physician's certification that they have less than six months to live. Smaller companies usually pay 50–80 percent of the benefit payable at death, although they will pay benefits to people who still have up to five years to live. The longer the person is expected to live, the less the cash disbursement.

Most insurers will not write new life insurance policies for persons known to have AIDS. However, the insurance industry has paid out more than $640 million in death benefits on policies of already-insured people who died of AIDS. At least one company does offer life insurance policies to some people infected with HIV, provided they meet certain eligibility requirements.

TREATMENT RESEARCH

Medical and pharmaceutical research to develop and conduct clinical trials of antiretroviral drugs is expensive. In 2002 the National Institutes of Health (NIH) will spend an estimated $2.5 billion for AIDS research, while spending about $630 million to investigate breast cancer, and $263 million for research about stroke.

Decisions about how much is spent to research a particular disease are not based solely on how many people develop the disease or die from it. Rightly or wrongly, economists base the societal value of an individual on his or her earning potential and productivity—the ability to contribute to society as a worker. The bulk of the people who die from heart disease, stroke, and cancer are older adults. Many have retired from the workforce, and their potential economic productivity is usually low or even nil. (This is not an observation about how society values older

TABLE 7.3

Ryan White CARE Act Title II grant awards, 1991–2000

STATE	FY 1991 - FY 1995	FY 1996 TOTAL	FY 1997 TOTAL	FY 1998 TOTAL	FY 1999 TOTAL	FY 2000 FORMULA	FY 2000 ADAP	FY 2000 TOTAL
ALABAMA	$4,829,350	$2,756,823	$4,167,971	$5,110,076	$7,294,833	$3,584,510	$4,639,040	$8,223,550
ALASKA	500,000	288,443	362,917	444,562	593,491	280,996	363,662	644,658
ARIZONA	5,707,125	2,260,259	3,496,214	4,553,503	6,281,940	2,639,155	5,237,395	7,876,550
ARKANSAS	2,819,849	1,369,814	2,050,008	2,505,494	3,313,331	1,625,526	2,103,741	3,729,267
CALIFORNIA	101,736,257	36,282,354	57,920,029	73,677,524	95,937,546	32,537,743	74,056,285	106,594,028
COLORADO	6,273,190	2,509,154	3,734,969	4,614,053	5,755,742	2,126,738	4,375,239	6,501,977
CONNECTICUT	7,398,150	3,651,778	6,120,430	8,267,209	11,422,933	3,778,961	8,694,101	12,473,062
DELAWARE	1,655,026	1,259,006	1,942,410	2,429,055	3,065,717	1,501,219	1,942,863	3,444,082
DIST. OF COLUMBIA	8,609,687	3,332,588	5,490,772	7,719,573	11,009,761	3,508,473	8,700,340	12,208,813
FLORIDA	62,624,900	25,220,349	41,314,996	53,845,136	73,482,287	27,331,222	56,820,710	84,151,932
GEORGIA	17,635,309	7,394,151	12,340,139	16,211,799	21,473,723	8,397,826	16,211,619	24,609,445
HAWAII	2,113,003	1,180,678	1,701,733	1,933,618	2,425,061	1,183,240	1,531,338	2,714,578
IDAHO	568,982	285,657	362,917	444,562	581,700	278,034	359,828	637,862
ILLINOIS	19,658,478	7,260,236	12,033,969	15,478,545	21,516,441	7,348,535	16,392,905	23,741,440
INDIANA	5,035,921	2,762,555	4,301,051	5,362,040	7,161,199	3,405,664	4,407,580	7,813,244
IOWA	1,157,658	613,264	917,406	1,104,116	1,450,320	696,217	901,037	1,597,254
KANSAS	2,000,328	1,050,840	1,565,364	1,888,481	2,407,272	1,049,083	1,631,556	2,680,639
KENTUCKY	2,458,912	1,344,978	2,078,323	2,882,026	4,075,831	2,039,702	2,639,763	4,679,465
LOUISIANA	10,104,144	4,080,447	6,969,329	9,199,630	13,072,061	5,384,296	9,275,299	14,659,595
MAINE	810,055	536,845	719,201	806,854	970,811	459,028	594,070	1,053,098
MARYLAND	14,021,974	6,521,685	10,948,524	14,847,982	20,672,553	7,081,339	16,544,049	23,625,388
MASSACHUSETTS	12,364,148	4,836,051	7,528,256	9,780,533	12,626,775	4,796,709	10,338,436	15,135,145
MICHIGAN	9,295,185	3,897,084	5,814,246	7,690,514	10,452,742	4,063,406	7,773,145	11,836,551
MINNESOTA	3,220,768	1,249,617	1,878,085	2,365,346	2,995,477	1,057,229	2,371,809	3,429,038
MISSISSIPPI	3,479,363	1,868,450	2,760,714	3,623,766	4,995,545	2,589,467	3,351,265	5,940,732
MISSOURI	9,053,788	3,131,126	4,586,448	5,952,010	7,811,393	2,899,468	5,943,296	8,842,764
MONTANA	456,197	129,912	201,037	375,524	477,324	250,000	243,995	493,995
NEBRASKA	923,095	506,277	733,358	931,421	1,206,634	594,386	769,249	1,363,635
NEVADA	3,194,245	2,049,946	3,001,392	3,898,380	4,647,952	1,598,090	3,364,738	4,962,828
NEW HAMPSHIRE	642,850	332,092	529,197	651,190	861,790	317,246	610,476	927,722
NEW JERSEY	29,042,291	13,135,111	21,380,789	28,345,926	37,702,846	12,815,241	27,947,200	40,762,441
NEW MEXICO	1,682,335	882,641	1,183,568	1,687,316	2,476,155	1,169,997	1,514,200	2,684,197
NEW YORK	103,550,023	38,324,520	64,354,160	87,884,362	127,095,837	42,636,690	95,825,514	138,462,204
NORTH CAROLINA	8,016,460	4,810,589	7,053,271	8,657,402	11,672,934	5,810,860	7,526,237	13,337,097
NORTH DAKOTA	419,872	107,243	124,390	145,189	175,060	100,000	83,474	183,474
OHIO	9,109,982	4,668,106	7,316,497	8,953,866	11,834,654	5,120,326	7,742,270	12,862,596
OKLAHOMA	3,581,484	1,656,387	2,282,191	2,890,518	3,902,893	1,867,782	2,417,266	4,285,048
OREGON	4,318,167	1,684,631	2,749,308	3,438,455	4,333,257	1,603,248	3,119,691	4,722,939
PENNSYLVANIA	17,227,187	7,991,467	12,944,947	16,937,810	23,632,455	9,309,084	17,587,661	26,896,745
RHODE ISLAND	1,585,172	1,083,242	1,548,831	1,843,025	2,354,312	1,122,008	1,452,093	2,574,101
SOUTH CAROLINA	7,019,356	4,516,376	6,622,883	8,161,966	10,934,388	5,775,847	7,475,048	13,250,895
SOUTH DAKOTA	500,000	112,536	138,843	161,507	205,084	101,714	131,638	233,352
TENNESSEE	5,770,766	3,757,915	5,736,623	7,230,546	9,818,153	4,998,883	6,469,509	11,468,392
TEXAS	44,589,664	16,132,517	25,697,515	35,149,403	50,244,224	18,736,047	38,195,998	56,932,045
UTAH	1,677,559	810,043	1,251,524	1,542,931	2,083,114	1,057,785	1,368,976	2,426,761
VERMONT	503,727	279,529	342,140	404,394	488,047	250,000	260,156	510,156
VIRGINIA	8,798,087	5,365,718	8,116,678	10,452,242	13,099,292	5,277,831	9,567,364	14,845,195
WASHINGTON	8,192,474	3,154,250	4,898,005	6,404,980	8,333,780	3,036,562	5,983,248	9,019,810
WEST VIRGINIA	774,743	446,290	740,356	937,140	1,422,541	616,555	846,071	1,462,626
WISCONSIN	3,429,155	1,840,433	2,579,528	3,054,537	3,812,983	1,847,729	2,394,773	4,242,502
WYOMING	444,037	113,650	137,940	169,038	196,506	100,000	105,536	205,536
GUAM	16,937	4,970	11,608	11,052	19,652	16,916	21,893	38,809
PUERTO RICO	31,723,832	9,376,181	12,920,475	16,793,353	23,401,013	8,248,605	17,399,027	25,647,632
VIRGIN ISLANDS	170,167	197,360	191,525	222,610	624,935	290,782	376,328	667,110
TOTALS	$612,491,414	$250,405,164	$397,895,000	$520,074,000	$709,904,300	$266,314,000	$528,000,000	$794,314,000

SOURCE: "Ryan White CARE Act Title II Grant Awards," in *Historical Funding Chart for Ryan White CARE Act*, Health Resources and Services Administration, Rockville, MD, January 2001 [Online] ftp://ftp.hrsa.gov/hab/fundinghistory.pdf [accessed December, 2001]

adults; instead it is simply an economic measure of present and future financial productivity.)

In contrast, AIDS patients are usually much younger, dying in their twenties, thirties, and forties. Until they developed AIDS their potential productivity, measured in economic terms, was high. The number of work years lost when they die is considerable. Using this economic equation to determine how disease research should be funded, it may be considered economically wise to invest more money to research AIDS since the losses, measured in potential work years rather than lives, is so much greater.

The primary goals of HIV/AIDS therapy are to prolong life and improve its quality. Few researchers expect any drug to cure HIV infection; their objective is to make the virus less deadly by foiling its efforts to reproduce within the body. A major obstacle to the discovery of such treatments is the cost of drug research and development. Pharmaceutical manufacturers spend millions of dollars researching and developing new medicines. According to the Pharmaceutical Research and Manufacturers of America, U.S. pharmaceutical companies spend more money each year on research and development activities than the annual budget of the NIH.(See Figure 7.1.)

A pharmaceutical manufacturer must cover the cost not only of research and development for the approximately 3 out of 10 drugs that succeed, but also for many—7 out of 10—that fail. Because of this cost, once a new drug receives FDA approval its manufacturer ordinarily holds a patent or gains exclusivity rights which guarantee it will be the sole marketer for a specified time (usually from 3 to 20 years) in order to recoup its investment. During that time, the drug is priced much higher than if other manufacturers were allowed to compete by producing generic versions of the same drug. In contrast to the original manufacturer, the generic manufacturer does not have to pay for successful and unsuccessful research and development of new drugs, nor does it have to pursue the complicated, time-consuming process of seeking FDA approval. The producer of generic drugs has the formula and must simply manufacture the drugs properly. Because of the lower cost of the generic drug after the original patent or exclusivity period has expired, competition between pharmaceutical manufacturers generally lowers the price. HIV/AIDS drugs are granted seven years of exclusivity under legislation aimed at encouraging research and promoting development of new treatments.

FDA-APPROVED DRUGS

The first drug thought to delay symptoms was zidovudine (earlier known as AZT, later as ZDV), but its effects have been found to be temporary at best. Several other drugs work on the same principle as ZDV, but until recently, it seemed that there was no way of stopping HIV. A new class of drugs called protease inhibitors (PI) appears to keep HIV already in the host cells from reproducing, unlike ZDV and similar drugs, which help keep HIV out of the cell's chromosomes. PIs block the ability of HIV to mature and infect new cells by suppressing a protein enzyme of the virus, called protease, which is crucial to the progression of HIV. One study conducted by Merck showed that a combination of Crixivan and two other AIDS drugs reduced virus load by more than 99 percent in patients with T cell counts between 50 and 400 per cubic millimeter. Another researcher, Dr. Keith Henry of Regions Hospital in St. Paul, Minnesota, found that PIs

reduced deaths by 85 percent in a selected HIV population under study.

Even if the effectiveness of PIs proves to be transient, they should improve patients' prospects simply by creating more roadblocks for HIV, which mutates so rapidly that it becomes resistant to most drugs when they are used alone. Even if a cure is never found, new and better drugs used in various combinations may make HIV infection a chronic, but manageable disease, much like diabetes.

The cost, however, is high. PIs range from about $4,800 to $8,000 for a year's supply. When combined with ZDV or any of the other commonly used antiretroviral drugs, such as lamivudine (3TC), zalcitabine (ddC), didanosine (ddI), or stavudine (d4T), the cost is approximately $18,000 per year. Government programs and private insurers alike are looking for ways to pay for, and in some cases, avoid paying for, these new therapies. As Moises Agosto of the National Minority AIDS Council in Washington, D.C., noted, though the drugs may be approved, people may still not be able to utilize the new treatments if programs can't afford them.

Types of Antiretroviral Agents

As of November 2001, the U.S. Food and Drug Administration (FDA) has accepted the following classes of antiretroviral agents for treatment of HIV/AIDS.

PROTEASE INHIBITORS (PIS). The following are protease inhibitors (PIs):

- Indinavir, manufactured by Merck, sold under brand name Crixivan (1996)

- Ritnavir, manufactured by Abbott, sold under brand name Norvir (1996)

- Saquinavir, manufactured by Hoffman-LaRoche, sold under brand name Invirase and Fortovase (1995)

- Nelfinavir, manufactured by Agouron, sold under brand name Viracept (1997)

- Amprenavir, manufactured by GlaxoSmithKline, sold under brand name Agenerase (1999)

Drugs formulated with combinations of two or more protease inhibitors also have received FDA approval:

- Lopinavir and Ritonavir, manufactured by Abbott Laboratories, sold under the brand name Kaletra (2000); for use in adult and pediatric patients

- Abacavir, Retrovir, and Lamivudine in a fixed dose combination, manufactured by GlaxoSmithKline, sold under the brand name Trizivir (2000)

NUCLEOSIDE ANALOGS. Nucleoside analogs limit HIV replication by incorporating themselves into a strand of DNA that causes the chain to end.

FIGURE 7.1

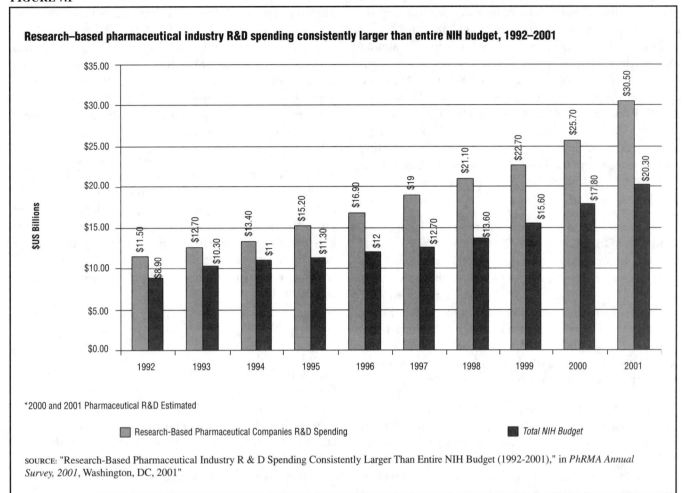

Research–based pharmaceutical industry R&D spending consistently larger than entire NIH budget, 1992–2001

*2000 and 2001 Pharmaceutical R&D Estimated

■ Research-Based Pharmaceutical Companies R&D Spending   ■ *Total NIH Budget*

SOURCE: "Research-Based Pharmaceutical Industry R & D Spending Consistently Larger Than Entire NIH Budget (1992-2001)," in *PhRMA Annual Survey, 2001*, Washington, DC, 2001"

- Zidovudine, manufactured by GlaxoSmithKline, sold under brand name Retrovir (1987)

- Didanosine, manufactured by Bristol-Myers Squibb, sold under brand name Videx (1991)

- Zalcitabine, manufactured by Hoffman-LaRoche, sold under brand name Hivid (1992)

- Stavudine, manufactured by Bristol Myers-Squibb, sold under brand name Zerit (1994)

- Lamivudine, manufactured by GlaxoSmithKline, sold under brand name Epivir (1995)

- Abacavir, manufactured by GlaxoSmithKline, sold under brand name Ziagen (1999)

NON-NUCLEOSIDE REVERSE TRANSCRIPTASE INHIB-ITORS (NNRTIS). Another class of antiretroviral drugs approved in the late 1990s is the non-nucleoside reverse transcriptase inhibitor (NNRTI). It slows down the process of the enzyme that allows the virus to become a part of the infected cell's nucleus. As of November 2001 there were three NNRTIs approved for use by the FDA:

- Nevirapine, manufactured by Boehringer Ingelheim Pharmaceuticals, sold under the brand name Viramune (1996)

- Delavirdine, manufactured by Pharmacia & Upjohn, sold under the brand name Rescriptor (1997)

- Efavirenz, manufactured by Dupont Pharmaceuticals, sold under the brand name Sustiva (1998)

NUCLEOTIDE ANALOGS. In October 2001 the FDA approved Viread (tenofovir disoproxil fumarate), the first nucleotide analog for HIV treatment. Nucleotide analogs are similar to nucleoside analogs in their action to block HIV replication. Intended for use in combination with other antiretroviral drugs, the new drug has been shown to reduce HIV replication; however, there are not yet long-term study results to demonstrate whether Viread effectively inhibits the clinical progression of HIV.

Aggressive Treatment

With new drugs in the anti-HIV/AIDS arsenal, where formerly only ZDV—a drug that was ineffective in the long run and had unpleasant side effects—existed, many people with HIV/AIDS who had given up hope of effective treatment returned to clinics and doctors' offices. While treatment guidelines previously promoted early intervention with ZDV, recommended treatment now combines PIs with other antiretroviral drugs. Treatment recommendations change rapidly in response to the development of new drugs and clinical trials indicating the effectiveness of different combinations of antiretroviral drugs. Researchers are acting quickly to develop new mixtures of the recently approved and older drugs. Because HIV mutates to resist any drug it faces, including all PIs, researchers have found that varying the combination of drugs prescribed can "fool" the virus before it has time to mutate.

Another approach to treatment, presented in an article published in the February 15, 2000 issue of the *Annals of Internal Medicine* by Keith Henry, M.D., suggested that overly aggressive antiretroviral therapy in the early stages of the disease may expose patients to unpleasant side effects and cause their systems to build resistance. Henry recommended a more cautious strategy: a long-term, patient-focused approach that would include delaying initial therapy; planned interruptions in drug dose administration; therapy switching; and immune-based therapy.

Patients undergoing therapy with these new drugs or drug combinations must be highly disciplined. For instance, Crixivan must be taken on an empty stomach, every eight hours, not less than two hours before or after a meal, and with large amounts of water to prevent development of kidney stones. Patients must also be careful to never skip doses of Crixivan; otherwise, HIV will quickly grow immune to its effect. (Crixivan has been found to generate cross-resistance, meaning it made patients resistant to other PIs.) Invirase must be taken in large doses. Norvir must be carefully prescribed and administered because it interacts negatively with some antifungals and antibiotics used by AIDS patients. Because there are a variety of minor and serious risks associated with use of these drugs, patients must be closely monitored.

The difficulty of dealing with a complicated regimen of daily medication has been an issue for HIV/AIDS patients. Dr. Henry argued that more support should be given to those health care professionals (such as nurses or pharmacists) who educate patients and assist them in maintaining their complicated daily medication schedules. During 2000 many combined HIV/AIDS medication regimens could be administered two to three times per day, and once-a-day regimens may be possible in the near future. Such a possibility, according to the researchers, would lead to improved adherence to treatment and quality of life for persons with HIV/AIDS.

LINGERING QUESTIONS. As observed earlier, the success of PIs may prove transient. Studies conducted by drug companies that produce the protease inhibitors have shown that viral loads decreased to undetectable levels for at least a few months whether the patients had been HIV-positive for a few weeks or a few years. Because the drugs were given the nod under the FDA's accelerated approval program—a fast-track approval after safety and efficacy are demonstrated in a single clinical trial—some investigators question their long-term efficacy. If each PI is able to suppress HIV for only a little while, critics ask, then are HIV/AIDS patients any better off?

Other questions persist. Even though patients with HIV treated with PIs may have no detectable HIV in their blood, might it still be present in their tissue? Will drug-resistant strains of the virus emerge over time? Will these powerful drugs cause harmful side effects if taken for long periods? Is it safe to switch from one drug to another once there's resistance? Studies are underway and more are planned to determine the optimal therapy and when it should begin.

THE DISCOVERY OF AN HIV-RESISTANT GENE

In August 1996 scientists working independently at the Aaron Diamond AIDS Research Center in New York City and the Free University of Brussels, Belgium, announced that some white people have genes that may protect them from HIV no matter how many times they are exposed to the virus. The researchers hope the findings could lead to new HIV/AIDS therapies or to the development of pills or injections to prevent HIV.

The gene, called CCR5 (CC chemokine receptor 5), is a mutant that fails to produce the protein that allows HIV to enter the surface of certain immune cells. The mutation causes the gene to have a hole in the middle of its DNA. Because of this, the CCR5 protein is deformed and the cell destroys it instead of displaying it on the surface as would be normal. Without the protein, HIV cannot invade the immune system. If a sex partner transmits HIV to a person with the CCR5 gene, the virus has nothing to which it can attach itself; therefore HIV appears to remain harmless.

Subsequent studies conducted in the U.S. found that 1 in 100 people inherits two copies of this gene—one from each parent—and is completely immune to HIV infection. The 1 in 5 people with only one copy of the CCR5 gene can become infected, but remains healthy two to three years longer than those without the altered gene. This may be because he or she has half as many CCR5 receptors as is normal, which limits or slows the spread of the virus.

Research studies in the United States found that the gene is most common in white Americans. It is found rarely in African Americans and almost never in Africans or Asians. Researchers speculate that the mutation occurred after the ancestors of today's Caucasians left Africa 100,000 years ago.

NEW RESEARCH

The Thymus Gland and the Immune System

One of the next major challenges in the fight against HIV/AIDS is reviving a deteriorated immune system. Without a healthy immune system, HIV/AIDS patients will not be able to recover from the disease, even if a cure is found. Researchers theorize that it may be possible to rejuvenate a wasted immune system. The key to this is the thymus gland, located next to the heart behind the breastbone. The thymus gland is where T cells mature. When mature, the T cells fight infections in the body. However, when HIV invades the body, the virus uses the T cell to replicate itself. The T cell does not survive this process, and the whole immune system collapses, leaving the HIV-infected patient susceptible to rare and often deadly infections.

Until the late 1990s it was thought that the thymus gland was only active during the first 30 years of life, and that no new T cells could be made thereafter. In recent years researchers have observed that the new drug combinations, often termed "cocktails," seem to be able to boost the number of T cells. No one, however, knows where these new cells are coming from. Currently doctors are using artificial means to increase the number of T cells in HIV-infected persons. However, if the adult body can indeed manufacture new T cells, it may be possible to restore the immune system.

"Morning After" Treatment

HIV has now been classified as a communicable sexually transmitted disease (STD) in the United States. A few doctors are beginning to prescribe some of the drugs used to treat established infections as "morning after" pills in an attempt to prevent transmission of the virus after risky sexual encounters. Currently, no studies show that this will work, and the medications are not licensed to be used this way, but other forms of HIV are halted by prompt use of the drugs, encouraging some doctors to give it a try. For example, an antiretroviral drug regimen given to hospital personnel following accidental needle stick from an HIV infected patient seems to reduce the one in 200 risk of transmission by about 80 percent. Similarly, antiretroviral treatment given to HIV-infected pregnant women reduces the risk of transmission to the newborn baby from one in four to less than one in ten.

This "off-label" use of potent PIs in an attempt to prevent the spread of HIV, however, is controversial. All drugs used in the treatment of HIV have side-effects, some of which may be potentially life threatening. Further, some researchers fear that if people believe "morning-after" treatment will prevent HIV infection they may stop taking precautions, such as using condoms, to prevent exposure to HIV. Others feel that the treatment is not appropriate as a preventive measure for persons exposed to ongoing risk, such as relationships where only one partner is infected, because the drugs are too toxic. Other methods such as the continued use of condoms would be much safer.

Finally, post-exposure treatment is expensive. The costs of two or three drugs taken for a month, plus laboratory tests and visits to the doctor, may run as high as $1,000. Of course this is a fraction of the cost for lifetime treatment of HIV infection and certainly money well spent if it prevents a person from acquiring the virus.

On the other hand, some researchers say that "morning after" treatment could save lives. The drugs, themselves, will save some lives, and the offer of treatment will bring people who are at high risk for acquiring HIV into environments where they can get counseling and care. In San Francisco, California, post-exposure treatment is offered to victims of rape as a matter of course. Some doctors feel that if the treatment does not work to prevent the disease, it may work to treat the disease. Though there is disagreement about the effectiveness and wisdom of widespread use of post-exposure treatment, nearly all researchers and health care providers agree that for sexually active people, the best prevention is the use of condoms.

Additional Research

There are several promising directions in HIV/AIDS treatment and research. Simplified medication regimens may improve adherence to treatment, and structured treatment interruptions allow the body to recover from the effects of medications. Structured treatment interruptions might, according to the theory, allow the body to regain immunity to HIV during breaks from the medication schedule. Other studies focus on better understanding HIV-specific immunity and how to retain or restore it, and research into nutritional deficiencies that might accelerate the disease among some patients.

IN SEARCH OF A VACCINE

Some pharmaceutical companies claim that because the of the high costs of research and development and the relatively low return on their investments, since the exclusivity period is limited to seven years, they have little financial incentive to develop new HIV/AIDS drugs. Likewise, they allege that they have little economic motivation to research and develop a vaccine for HIV. In February 1996 Dr. Anthony Fauci, head of the National Institute of Allergy and Infectious Diseases (NIAID), released guidelines to promote cooperation between the government and private industry. The plan's goal is to overcome the alleged unfavorable market forces that have caused some companies to abandon research of potential HIV vaccines.

Executives of pharmaceutical and biotechnology companies believe that government officials arbitrarily change the rules when deciding to move vaccine trials from one stage of testing to the next. Dr. Fauci's guidelines, which were endorsed by the FDA, detail the path for vaccine testing and the criteria that must be met before a vaccine trial can move on to successive stages.

There are problems of experimental design and ethical considerations involved in vaccine trials using human volunteers. Most volunteers for the vaccine have behaviors that put them at risk for contracting HIV. Some volunteers may mistakenly believe that participating in the clinical trial of an experimental vaccine—which may be vaccine or placebo—protects them and, with a false sense of security, they may resume high-risk behaviors.

If these volunteers contract HIV during the clinical trial, then scientists cannot be sure whether it is from risky behaviors or from the experimental vaccine (some vaccines may contain live HIV because a weakened version of the virus itself is used to stimulate the body's immune system to act against the virus). When volunteers contract HIV during trials, the testing is abandoned. On the other hand, volunteers may reduce their risks so successfully that they are never exposed to HIV, leaving the vaccine nothing to fight. This paradox is unique to HIV/AIDS research and frustrates scientists.

Despite optimistic projections in the early 1990s that a vaccine would be found by 1995, a considerable number of promising experimental HIV vaccines have proven ineffective against strains of HIV taken from infected people. Researchers have reported developing antibodies that worked successfully against HIV grown in test tubes, but in every case they failed when used against HIV in actual human beings. NIAID's Dr. Fauci commented that the results of initial vaccine research were "cause for some sober reflection."

Robert Gallo, one of the co-discoverers of HIV and the director of the Institute of Human Virology at the University of Maryland in Baltimore, is cautiously optimistic about the development of the HIV vaccine. Speaking at the first World Congress on Men's Health in Vienna, Austria in October 2001, he predicted that one of the vaccines currently under investigation would likely be successful. Gallo said he believes an effective HIV vaccine is "realistically at least five years away."

The First Large-Scale Human Test

In June 1998 the FDA gave VaxGen, Inc., of San Francisco, California, permission to conduct the world's first full-scale test of a vaccine to prevent HIV infection. The VaxGen vaccine had been found safe in tests involving 1,200 volunteers in March 1992, with more than 99 percent of the vaccinated participants producing antibodies. The 1998 test involved 5,000 volunteers in 40 clinics throughout the U.S. and Canada, and 2,500 volunteers in

16 clinics in Thailand. The largest human study of an HIV vaccine to date, the four-year trial ends in 2002.

Three injections of the genetically engineered vaccine Aidsvax were given to volunteers over several months. The vaccine is made from part of HIV's outer coat, known as gp120, which attaches to cells to infect them. The vaccine does not cause the disease because it is made from a tiny amount of viral protein from two strains of HIV. (Previous vaccines used one strain.) The two strains of the vaccine that were tested in North America are made with strains common in North America; the vaccine used in Thailand contained strains common to that part of the world. Participants in the North American study were men who have sex with men and uninfected partners of HIV-positive people. In Thailand, volunteers were uninfected injecting drug users (IDUs). Two-thirds of the North American volunteers were given the vaccine, and the rest received a placebo. In Thailand, half the group received the vaccine and half were given a placebo.

Although health officials and AIDS activists are hopeful, scientists are divided over when and which experimental vaccines should be approved for full-scale testing. Some favor trying any promising vaccine, others advise waiting until the vaccine is completely understood before testing it. The results of the clinical trial will be analyzed in an attempt to determine how effective the experimental vaccine is against development of HIV in people exposed to the virus through high-risk sexual practices or injected drug use.

One problem with the vaccine is that previous tests indicated that it boosted only one part of the immune system involving antibodies. Most experts believe that an anti-HIV vaccine must boost another part of the immune system—the killer T cells that destroy virus-infected cells. Some experts consider the vaccine a long shot, but others point out that a failed vaccine does not mean that the experiment failed. Negative results can teach researchers what not to do in the future.

Since clinical trials began for the first vaccine targeting HIV, more than 30 additional studies of other HIV vaccines have begun. In 2000 the Dale and Betty Bumpers Vaccine Research Center (VRC) opened on the NIH campus in Bethesda, Maryland. The $34 million facility is overseen by Anthony Fauci, M.D., director of the National Institute of Allergy and Infectious Diseases and brings together private companies and federal agencies to research, develop, and produce vaccines. Though VRC is not exclusively devoted to HIV research, and will eventually begin efforts to develop vaccines for other diseases, VRC director Gary Nabel says HIV is a first target for the new facility, which has $40 million in funding for 2002.

The first testing at VRC began in October 2001 and is a study of VRC-001-VP, a DNA vaccine that contains tiny amounts of re-engineered HIV DNA. The clinical trial of VRC-001-VP involves volunteers who are not necessarily at risk for HIV infection and seeks to answer questions about how the immune system responds to the vaccine and the best timing for administering second and third doses of the vaccine.

While most researchers are optimistic that an effective vaccine will be developed, many believe it may take as long as ten years to perfect a vaccine. Currently, researchers at the VRC believe that more than one vaccine formulation, or a vaccine that works two ways—to boost immunity provided by T cells and produce antibodies to attach to HIV and mark it for destruction—may be necessary to provide complete protection.

A Dissenting View on Why There Is No Vaccine

A small group of researchers who call themselves the Group for the Scientific Reappraisal of the HIV-AIDS Hypothesis dispute that AIDS is caused by HIV, the view widely held by the rest of the world's scientific community. Peter Duesberg, a professor of molecular and cell biology at the University of California at Berkeley and discoverer of the first cancer-related gene in 1970, and Kary Mullis, winner of the 1993 Nobel Prize in chemistry, believe that HIV does not cause AIDS. (The two disagree on exactly what causes the disease, but they do agree that HIV is *not* the cause.) In *Inventing the AIDS Virus* (Regnery, 1996) Duesberg observes that despite huge efforts—over 100,000 research papers published and $35 billion in taxpayer dollars spent—the HIV/AIDS hypothesis has failed to produce any public-health benefits.

Duesberg bases his hotly disputed, highly controversial hypothesis, in part, on the fact that existing theories concerning the cause of AIDS rely on epidemiological, or circumstantial, evidence—that HIV is found in all persons who have AIDS—and not scientific proof that directly connects HIV and AIDS. If an infectious agent caused AIDS, Duesberg explains, it would exhibit five distinct qualities:

1. It would spread randomly between the sexes.

2. AIDS would appear quickly, in a matter of weeks or months instead of years.

3. Active and plentiful HIV microbes would be identifiable in all cases.

4. Cells would decrease or be impaired to the extent that the immune system could not replace them.

5. There would be a logical and consistent pattern of symptoms in AIDS patients.

His reasoning is compelling to some: none of the above qualities has been observed with HIV. Infection among men is far more common than in women, though this is changing; the onset of AIDS can take up to 11 years; the virus is difficult to isolate; cells in AIDS patients are replaced; and symptoms vary among patients.

Duesberg's critics contend that the overwhelming body of research links HIV to AIDS. Even some of Duesberg's critics, however, still agree with his basic observation: because more than 20 years have passed since AIDS was first described, and research has failed to substantially change the fate of people with HIV/AIDS, new paths of investigation may be in order.

CHAPTER 8
PEOPLE WITH HIV/AIDS

Given the staggeringly large numbers of persons with HIV/AIDS in the U.S. and the increasing proportion of people living with HIV infection, Americans are now, more than ever before, likely to know someone affected by HIV/AIDS. Even people who live in remote geographic areas and do not believe they are personally at risk of acquiring HIV are aware of the epidemic from ongoing public health education campaigns, reports in the media, school health programs, and health and social service agencies dedicated to improving community awareness of HIV/AIDS.

CELEBRITIES WITH HIV/AIDS

Perhaps one of the most famous HIV-infected persons in the world is Earvin "Magic" Johnson, internationally known former basketball player for the Los Angeles Lakers. When Johnson announced his HIV infection in September 1991, the world was shocked. He had no idea he was infected until he received the results of a routine physical examination for life insurance. Johnson freely admitted that prior to his marriage he had unprotected, and as such unsafe, sexual contact with numerous women and had no idea who had transmitted the virus to him.

To many, Johnson became a hero for his courage and his immediate public acknowledgment of his HIV status. He became an HIV/AIDS spokesman and began working in prevention programs. In 1991 Johnson started the Magic Johnson Foundation, which seeks to find funding and establish community-based education, social, and health programs (including HIV/AIDS awareness) in inner-city communities and has given millions of dollars in grants to these causes. He was even named to the President's Commission on AIDS, from which he eventually resigned. Despite his active, well-publicized efforts to increase awareness and prevention of HIV/AIDS, some people considered him anything but a hero because his highly visible, promiscuous lifestyle sent the wrong message to the millions of young people who admired him.

In September 1992, one year after Johnson announced his retirement from professional basketball, he indicated that he was returning to basketball on a limited basis. He played on the United States "Dream Team" in the 1992 Olympics, assisting the team in its successful bid for the Gold Medal. Johnson benched himself at the start of the 1993–94 season when he cut himself in a pre-season game, terrifying some of his fellow players. While some players feared infection, others worried that they should not play against Johnson with full force; after all, he was a man with a fatal disease. Johnson came back again for the 1995–96 season, helping his team reach the playoffs, and continues to play basketball with the Magic Johnson All Stars Team. He has shown others, as one observer noted, that HIV infection is not something you die with; it is something you live with.

In 1992 former tennis star Arthur Ashe announced that he had become infected with HIV from a blood transfusion in the mid-1980s during a heart bypass operation. His was not a voluntary announcement, but one made necessary when the news media discovered his HIV infection and threatened to announce it before he did. Ashe was reluctant to make his condition public, fearing the effect on his five-year-old daughter. He maintained that because he did not have a public responsibility he should have been allowed to maintain his privacy. He died in 1994.

Another athlete, Greg Louganis, was diagnosed with HIV infection in 1988. The Olympic gold-medalist diver announced his HIV status after the 1992 Olympics, when he hit his head on the diving board during competition. Though his injury was not serious, it did result in an open wound. Today Louganis is a television and movie actor, the published author of two books, and an advocate of safe sexual practices, since he attributes his HIV infection to unsafe sexual behavior.

Mary Fisher, a heterosexual and non-drug-user who contracted HIV from her husband, stood before her peers at the 1992 Republican Convention and announced that she was infected with HIV. A former television producer and assistant to President Gerald R. Ford, she said she considered her announcement part of her contribution to the fight against HIV/AIDS. The wealthy, attractive, and well-educated Fisher was among the first women to publicly dispel the image that usually comes to mind when most people think of HIV/AIDS—homosexual, poor, drug-addicted, and lacking access to support systems or adequate medical care and housing.

OLDER PEOPLE WITH HIV/AIDS

The CDC, in *Morbidity and Mortality Weekly Report* ("AIDS Among Persons Aged 50 Years and Over—United States, 1991–1996," Vol. 47, No. 2, 1998), reported that most older people infected with HIV early in the epidemic were typically infected through contaminated blood or blood products. Through 1989 only 1 percent of cases of persons with HIV/AIDS ages 13–49 was due to contaminated blood. However, in that same period, 6 percent of cases of persons 50–59, 28 percent of cases of persons 60–69, and 64 percent of cases of those 70 and older resulted from contaminated blood or blood products.

In 1985 changes introduced to improve the safety of the nation's blood, including routine screening of blood donations for HIV, sharply reduced the risk of contracting the virus from contaminated blood or blood products. Subsequently, the proportion of those aged 50 and over acquiring HIV from other types of exposure increased. Although MSM contact and injection drug use (IDU) remain the primary means by which HIV is transmitted among all age groups in the U.S., heterosexual transmission of HIV is steadily increasing in persons more than 50 years old.

HIV/AIDS Cases Among Persons Age 50 and Over

Approximately 11–15 percent of AIDS cases reported in the U.S. occur in persons over age 50. This proportion did not vary much between 1991 and 1999. However, it is expected to increase as HIV-infected people of all ages live longer as a result of effective drug therapy and other advances in medical treatment.

From when record-keeping began to December 2000, 84,044 cases of AIDS in persons over age 50 were reported to the CDC. Among these reported cases 15 percent were women and 55 percent were persons of color (non-white). (See Table 3.6 in Chapter 3.) More than three-quarters of AIDS cases reported in persons over age 65 were from large metropolitan areas.

HIV Testing for Those Over 50

Many older adults do not seek routine screening for HIV infection because they do not believe they are at risk of acquiring HIV. Among women, the absence of the risk of pregnancy may lead to a false sense of security and the mistaken belief that they are at less risk for sexually transmitted diseases including HIV. HIV-infected persons age 50 and over may not be tested promptly for HIV infection, and as a result, opportunities to start these patients on therapies quickly in order to slow the progression of the disease are often lost. The failure to test or the late testing of older patients may be because:

- Physicians are less apt to look for HIV in persons of this age group.
- Some AIDS opportunistic illnesses (OIs) that occur in older persons, such as encephalopathy and wasting disease, have similar symptoms to other diseases associated with aging, such as Alzheimer's disease, depression, and malignancies.

It is vitally important to overcome older adults' reluctance to seek testing and other delays to diagnosis because recent research shows that age speeds the progression of HIV to AIDS and blunts CD4 response to highly active antiretroviral therapy (HAART). Equally important is continuing research to improve treatment of HIV-infected older adults and development of effective education programs to prevent infection in this population.

EMOTIONAL PROBLEMS

In order to gain a more complete view of the impact of HIV/AIDS, it is important to understand the psychosocial and emotional consequences of diagnosis with a potentially fatal disease.

A Frightening Diagnosis

In his introduction to *When Someone Close Has AIDS* (National Institute of Mental Health, Washington, D.C., 1989) NIMH director Dr. Lewis L. Judd wrote about the meaning of the diagnosis of AIDS. It means not only a shortened life, but also one that is "marred by chronic fatigue, loss of appetite and weight, frequent hospitalizations, AIDS dementia, and debilitating bouts of illness from unusual infections." The person diagnosed with HIV/AIDS also feels anger, confusion, depression, isolation, and hopelessness, which can also affect those around him or her who are often unprepared for the suffering they witness.

Dr. Judd advised that people diagnosed with HIV/AIDS need reassurance from friends and relatives that they will not be abandoned or isolated. He also recommended that those around HIV/AIDS patients encourage them to pursue hobbies, work as long as they can, and engage in social activities. He warned that caring for someone with AIDS is physically and emotionally exhausting and calls for inner strength as well as the caregivers' coming to terms with their own feelings about the illness.

Living with HIV/AIDS

COPING WITH DISCRIMINATION. Unlike people diagnosed with other terminal or catastrophic illnesses such as cancer or multiple sclerosis, people with HIV/AIDS often confront the social isolation and discrimination that accompanies a stigmatized status. Many people think of HIV/AIDS as a disease of men who have sex with men and drug users and believe that these people brought HIV/AIDS upon themselves. Fear of unfavorable judgment keeps many infected individuals from disclosing their HIV infection to others, even friends and loved ones. Others simply do not want the pity that is often extended to people with fatal conditions. Still others worry that friends and family, fearing infection, will abandon them.

Under the Americans with Disabilities Act of 1990 (ADA), persons infected with HIV and those diagnosed with AIDS are considered disabled and as such are subject to the anti-discrimination provisions of this landmark legislation. As a result, employers generally may not ask job applicants if they are HIV-infected or have AIDS, nor can they require an HIV test of prospective employees. The only exceptions to this provision are those employers that can demonstrate that such questions or testing are job-related and absolutely necessary for the employer to conduct business.

More importantly, the ADA requires employers to make "reasonable accommodations" for disabled employees. Reasonable accommodation is an adjustment to a job or modification of the responsibilities or work environment that will enable the worker with a disability to gain equal employment opportunity. Examples of reasonable accommodations employers have made for HIV-infected workers include flexible work schedules to allow them to attend medical appointments and receive treatment and counseling, and provision of additional unpaid leave.

THE STIGMA OF AIDS. In 1995 the Department of Sociology and Social Work at Fort Hays State University, Kansas, conducted a survey to find how knowledge and mode of transmission affected opinions of Persons With AIDS. J. J. Leiker, D. E. Taub, and J. Gast, in "The Stigma of AIDS: Persons with AIDS and Social Distance" (*Deviant Behavior*, October–December 1995), wrote that as HIV/AIDS knowledge increases, people tend to attach less stigma to the disease.

According to the survey, respondents attached the least stigma to those infected by blood transfusions. The greatest stigma was attached to exposures from MSM and IDU. Survey participants who considered themselves homophobic (having a fear of or aversion to homosexuality) attached more stigma to persons with AIDS than those who did not feel they were homophobic. People who labeled themselves "religious" attached less stigma to those infected through blood transfusions.

More than two decades after the first diagnoses of AIDS and widespread public health and community education efforts to inform people about HIV infection and prevent the spread of HIV, ignorance and misunderstanding of HIV/AIDS persist. Health educators and HIV/AIDS activists stress the importance of intensified, ongoing education to destigmatize persons affected by HIV/AIDS and prevent discrimination. Reducing the stigma associated with HIV/AIDS also may encourage individuals to get tested and, for those who are infected, begin treatment as soon as possible.

An article written by Rebecca Voelker, "Will Focus on Terrorism Overshadow the Fight Against AIDS?" in the *Journal of the American Medical Association* (November 7, 2001) observes that after more than two decades, the stigma associated with AIDS should have dropped to very low, barely detectable levels. Unfortunately, it has not diminished as expected. Researcher Lisanne Francis Brown of Tulane University School of Public Health feels it is important to identify strategies to reduce stigma since "stigma undermines efforts to combat the epidemic at every level."

DEALING WITH EMOTIONS. Not unexpectedly, anger and depression are natural and common reactions to discovering that one has an HIV infection. While experts stress the importance of recognizing and expressing anger and depression, if these feelings become all-consuming, they can prevent health- and life-improving actions. Many persons with HIV/AIDS admit that sharing feelings with friends, and family members and participating in support groups ease anguish and help to generate more positive attitudes and actions.

Many HIV/AIDS sufferers report that the most difficult thing they had to do after being diagnosed with HIV was to inform people in their present or recent past whom they might have exposed to the virus. If the patient is unable to do this, a physician or public health official can notify present or former sexual partners without revealing the infected person's name.

EARLY MEDICATION IMPROVES OUTLOOK. The earlier a person learns of his or her infection, the earlier he or she can begin medical treatment to suppress the virus's destructive growth, delay the onset of AIDS symptoms, and extend life. Along with antiretroviral drugs there are medications that fight the life-threatening opportunistic infections that eventually afflict most persons who are HIV-infected. Although these drugs cannot cure HIV infection, they have been shown to keep HIV/AIDS patients healthy and symptom-free for increasingly longer periods.

PRACTICING GOOD HEALTH HABITS. Experts advise HIV-infected persons to exercise and maintain a balanced diet with sufficient lean protein. Not only does exercise improve overall fitness and sense of well-being, it also releases endorphins, natural substances produced by the brain that boost immunity, reduce stress, and elevate mood. Persons with HIV/AIDS are advised to avoid smoking, illegal drugs, and excessive alcohol drinking, all of which can act to depress the immune system.

STRESS NOT A FACTOR? In addition to new health concerns, persons with HIV/AIDS must confront an altered identity. Instead of being seemingly healthy, those diagnosed with HIV infection are instantly transformed into people who must re-evaluate their goals—saving money for retirement or a new car may no longer seem important. HIV-infected individuals often lose their health insurance coverage and must consider saving money for future health care needs and/or meeting eligibility requirements for health care coverage from Medicaid, the government entitlement program. They also must confront fears and uncertainty about the future such as how to care and provide for children or other loved ones.

Interestingly, a study conducted by Ronald C. Kessler, research scientist at the University of Michigan's Institute for Social Research, indicated that stressful life events do not appear to trigger the development of AIDS symptoms in HIV-positive men who are feeling healthy. The findings, released in 1992, were based on correlation between the health and psychological status of 980 gay men in Chicago who participated in two studies from 1984 to 1987 (*The National Multicenter AIDS Cohort Study* and the *Coping and Change Study*, both funded by the National Institute of Mental Health). The results of this landmark study were considered to conclusively refute the hypothesis that stress plays a pivotal role in triggering the development of AIDS among persons with HIV infection.

The data, collected twice each year, included the incidence and nature of stressful life events and the development of three HIV symptoms—fevers lasting longer than two weeks, bacterial infections of the throat and mouth (oral thrush), and declines of 25 percent or more in the number of T cells. One aim of the study was to investigate the findings of an earlier unpublished study that had found HIV-positive men who were close to others with AIDS or persons dying from AIDS often experienced a sudden onset of symptoms themselves.

The University of Michigan study measured the impact of 24 other serious stresses on health, such as job loss, death of a parent, and mortgage foreclosure, and found no consistent relationship between stressful events and the onset of HIV symptoms. Kessler did find that men who were grieving for deceased loved ones were more likely to suffer a decline in T cells and develop other symptoms, but he did not believe that this was an effect of a stressful event. Instead, it is more likely that those who had an onset of symptoms after friends died from AIDS were probably in the same group who were infected early in the epidemic.

HOUSING PROBLEMS

The difficulty in finding affordable and appropriate housing can be an acute crisis for persons living with HIV/AIDS. HIV-infected persons need more than just a safe shelter that provides protection and comfort; they also may require a base from which to receive services, care, and support. While adherence to complicated medical regimens is challenging for many HIV-infected people, for some homeless people it is nearly impossible.

While some individuals are homeless when they acquire HIV infection, others lose their homes when they are no longer able to hold jobs or cannot afford to pay for health care and housing costs. According to 1999 reports from the National Coalition for the Homeless, an estimated 3–20 percent of the homeless are infected with HIV, and the number is growing daily. The CDC reported that some health care sites have reported HIV prevalence rates as high as 21.4 percent among selected homeless populations in the United States.

The Department of Veteran Affairs has reported that as many as one-third to one-half of all persons with HIV/AIDS are either homeless or at great risk of becoming homeless due to their illness, lack of income or other resources, and weak support networks. Several studies have indicated that approximately 30 percent of all persons with HIV in acute care hospitals (at a cost of more than $1,000 per day) are hospitalized not because they require the acute medical services available in the hospital, but simply because no community-based residential program will take them. According to the National Coalition for the Homeless, 1999 data showed that more than 30 percent of HIV-infected people had become homeless since learning they were infected. The same data predicted that 50 percent of people living with HIV/AIDS would need housing assistance during their lifetimes.

In 1990 the Department of Housing and Urban Development (HUD) established a federal program specifically intended to meet the housing needs of people with HIV/AIDS. Congress established the program because the housing resources available at that time were not meeting the needs of people with AIDS, who, due to discrimination, had difficulties obtaining suitable housing and the supportive services that they required. The program, Housing Opportunities for Persons With AIDS (HOPWA), was established under the National Affordable Housing Act of 1990 (PL 101-625). HOPWA began in 1992, and between that fiscal year (FY) and FY 2001, Congress allotted more than $1.5 billion for the program. In FY 2002 an additional $277 million was allocated, an increase of $19 million over the preceding year.

SUICIDE

Depression is a common psychiatric problem among patients who are seriously ill with HIV/AIDS. While this is a normal grief response, the combination of feelings of alienation, hopelessness, guilt, and lack of self-esteem can lead some to contemplate and plan for suicide in search of lost dignity and control. Others counter that the real dignity is in seeing the disease to the end. Those who encourage people with HIV/AIDS to "stick it out" often see the disease as becoming increasingly manageable with drugs and improved treatment techniques.

Several factors make HIV/AIDS patients more likely to commit suicide: they know they are certain to die sooner than they expected, and chances are it will be emotionally and physically painful; they may lose their jobs, their insurance, or their homes; and they may be ostracized from society. Researchers have found that factors with considerable impact on the quality of life include security, family, love, pleasurable activity, and freedom from pain and suffering and from debilitating disease. AIDS patients may lose all of these. For some, suicide is an apparently attractive alternative; it offers an end to pain and suffering, insecurity, self-pity, dependency, and hopelessness.

Euthanasia (ending the lives, for reasons of mercy, of those who are hopelessly ill or injured) and physician-assisted suicide are other unnatural deaths that are often requested by patients themselves. A 1995 study sponsored by Amsterdam's Municipal Health Service found that 22 percent of 131 men with AIDS that they studied died from requested euthanasia or physician-assisted suicide. Among the 22 percent, physicians reported that 72 percent would have died within one month. The survey also found that the likelihood of euthanasia/physician-assisted suicide increased with the duration of survival after AIDS diagnosis and among those over the age of 40.

The authors of the Amsterdam study noted that because AIDS patients usually know for many years that they are infected with HIV, they have time to discuss their condition and the possibility of euthanasia. Though technically illegal in the Netherlands, euthanasia is considered permissible when repeatedly requested by lucid patients who suffer from unbearable and incurable pain. Many of these people, explained a counselor of AIDS patients, choose euthanasia because it gives them the opportunity to die on their own terms.

The Physicians' Role

In 1994–95, Lee R. Slome, et al. ("Physician-Assisted Suicide and Patients with Human Immunodeficiency Virus Disease," *The New England Journal of Medicine*, Vol. 336, No. 6, 1997) surveyed all 228 physicians in the Community Consortium in the San Francisco Bay area of California. The researchers wanted to find out whether physicians were participating—or would be willing to participate to any extent—in physician-assisted suicide, which was defined as providing a patient with a sufficient dose of narcotics to kill himself or herself.

The physicians, who treated HIV patients, were told in the anonymous, self-administered survey that the ficti-

TABLE 8.1

Characteristics of physicians given physician-assisted suicide with HIV survey

Characteristic	1990 (N=69)	1995 (N=118)
	percent	
Sex		
Male	81	73
Female	19	27
Race or ethnic group[1]		
White	97	89
Black	0	4
Hispanic	1	3
Asian or Pacific Islander	2	4
Sexual orientation[2]		
Homosexual or bisexual	55	36
Heterosexual	45	64
Marital status		
Married	33	47
Unmarried but in a relationship	36	32
Unmarried and not in a relationship	30	21
Religion		
Protestant	26	17
Catholic	13	12
Jewish	36	30
Other	25	41
Total no. of patients with AIDS[3]		
0	9	0
1-20	4	3
21-40	7	8
41-60	7	4
61-80	9	5
>80	63	78

[1]P=0.05 for the comparison of the relative proportions of white and nonwhite respondents in the two surveys.
[2]P=0.01 for the comparison between the two surveys.
[3]P=0.01 for the comparison of the distribution of numbers of patients between the two surveys. Because of rounding, percentages do not sum to 100.

SOURCE: Lee R. Slome, Thomas F. Mitchell, Edwin Charlebois, et al., "Characteristics of Respondents to the 1990 and 1995 Surveys," in "Physician Assisted-Suicide and Patients with Human Immunodeficiency Virus Disease," *The New England Journal of Medicine*, vol. 336, no. 6, February 6, 1997

tious patient, Tom, was a severely ill, mentally incompetent 30-year-old man facing imminent death. A similar survey had been conducted in 1990. Compared with the 1990 respondents, the 118 physicians who responded to the 1995 survey were more racially diverse, more likely to be heterosexual, and more apt to have a large number of AIDS patients. (See Table 8.1.)

Of the 1995 respondents, 48 percent said they would be likely or very likely to grant Tom's initial request for physician-assisted suicide, compared with 28 percent of the 1990 respondents. When asked what they would do if Tom was adamant (insistent) about his request, 51 percent of the 1995 respondents said they would grant Tom's request, compared with 35 percent of the 1990 respondents. The 1995 physicians (11 percent) were also less likely than the 1990 physicians (23 percent) to try to talk the patient out of his request. (See Table 8.2.)

Slome and his colleagues also asked the physician respondents to estimate the number of times they had

TABLE 8.2

Physician responses to case vignette in 1990–95

Question and Response	1990	1995
	no. (%)	
How likely would you be to prescribe a lethal dose of medication for Tom?[1]		
Very unlikely	20 (29)	18 (16)
Unlikely	20 (29)	19 (17)
Neither likely nor unlikely	9 (13)	22 (19)
Likely	13 (19)	47 (41)
Very likely	6 (9)	8 (7)
If Tom was adamant about getting assistance in committing suicide, what course of action would you take?[2]		
Refuse his request	10 (14)	18 (16)
Talk him out of it[3]	16 (23)	12 (11)
Hospitalize him as a danger to himself	2 (3)	1 (1)
Refer him to a mental health professional	41 (59)	50 (45)
Refer him to a suicide-prevention program	4 (6)	5 (5)
Refer him to clergy	11 (16)	17 (15)
Refer him to another physician	1 (1)	8 (7)
Refer him to the Hemlock Society	32 (46)	42 (38)
Grant his request[4]	24 (35)	56 (51)

Note: Only the physicians who responded to question about the case vignette are included.
[1]There were 68 respondents in 1990 and 114 in 1995. P=0.005 for the comparison of the distribution of responses between the two surveys.
[2]There were 69 respondents in 1990 and 110 in 1995. More than one response per physician was possible.
[3]P=0.04 for the comparison of the distribution of responses between the two surveys.
[4]P=0.05 for the comparison of the distribution of responses between the two surveys.

SOURCE: Lee R. Slome, Thomas F. Mitchell, Edwin Charlebois, et al., "Responses to the Case Vignette in 1990 and 1995," in "Physician-Assisted Suicide and Patients with Human Immunodeficiency Virus Disease," *The New England Journal of Medicine*, vol. 336, no. 6, February 6, 1997

FIGURE 8.1

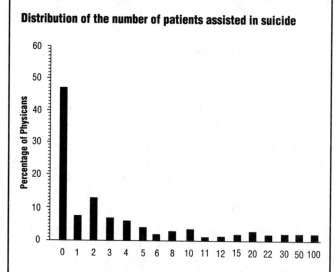

Distribution of the number of patients assisted in suicide

SOURCE: Lee R. Slome, Thomas F. Mitchell, Edwin Charlebois, et al., Distribution of the Number of Patients Assisted in Suicide, as Reported by 117 Physician Respondents to the 1995 Survey," in "Physician-Assisted Suicide and Patients with Human Immunodeficiency Virus Disease," *The New England Journal of Medicine*, vol. 336, no. 6, February 6, 1997.

helped an AIDS patient commit suicide. Of the 117 who responded, about half (52 percent) indicated that they had prescribed a fatal dose of medication at least once to an AIDS patient. (Figure 8.1 shows the distribution of the number of patients assisted in suicide.) The researchers noted that this number was surprisingly high, given the possible legal and ethical consequences of such an action.

Finally, the researchers concluded that:

• The survey suggests an increasing acceptance among physicians of assisted suicide.

• A physician's sexual orientation (homosexual or bisexual) is positively related to his or her willingness to assist in suicide, although sexual orientation is only one of four factors affecting the doctors' decision. (See Table 8.1 for other factors or characteristics of respondents.)

• Some doctors consider their assistance psychological intervention rather than a means of facilitating death; that is, the medication allows patients to regain some of the control AIDS has taken away.

During the 1990s there were heated debates, voter initiatives, and court decisions about the legalization of physician-assisted suicide. Only one U.S. state—Oregon—has legalized physician-assisted suicide; Oregon voters determined that the right to end one's own life is intensely personal and should not be forbidden by law. (Though attempts and acts of suicide are no longer subject to criminal prosecution in the U.S., aiding of suicide is considered a criminal offense.)

Both the public and physicians themselves are divided about the issue of physician-assisted suicide. People who support the practice believe that doctors should make their skills available to patients to end anguish and suffering. Those who oppose physician-assisted suicide argue that better end-of-life-care—effective pain management, emotional and spiritual support, and widespread education to reduce anxiety about dying—may reduce the frequency of requests for euthanasia. Opponents also fear that the legal right to assist suicide has the potential to be misused or abused, and that such abuses might victimize already vulnerable populations.

CHAPTER 9
TESTING, PREVENTION, AND EDUCATION

Every case must be located, reported, its source ascertained and all contacts then informed about the possibility of infection and, if infected, treated.

— Thomas Parran, director of the nation's anti-venereal-disease program, talking about sexually transmitted diseases in 1936

HIV TESTING

Voluntary, Not Mandatory

Few issues about the HIV/AIDS epidemic have prompted more controversy than the use of antibody tests to identify persons who are infected with HIV. Soon after the enzyme-linked immunosorbent assay (ELISA) test was developed and licensed in 1985, many public health officials supported testing in an attempt to change "undesirable" behaviors that were determining the course of the epidemic (e.g., MSM behavior and injected drug abuse). Those who favored testing claimed that, if a person knew he or she was HIV-positive, the infected person would change his or her behavior. Others argued that aggressive public health education and carefully planned and implemented counseling would be more productive strategies to achieve the desired results, even if persons did not know their HIV status.

In the early years of the epidemic, health care officials in the public and private sectors refrained from advocating mandatory testing, instead focusing on HIV testing that would be performed by physicians for patients they believed to be at risk for infection. In 1990 the House of Delegates of the American Medical Association (AMA) voted to declare HIV/AIDS a sexually transmitted disease (STD). With HIV/AIDS considered an STD, physicians were freer to decide the conditions under which HIV testing should take place.

In the late 1980s, when the research community announced that HIV-infected, symptom-free persons could receive early intervention with AZT (zidovudine, now known as ZDV) to slow the effects of the illness and delay the onset of *Pneumocystis carinii* pneumonia (PCP), the debate took another turn. Gay rights advocates, such as the Gay Men's Health Crisis Center in New York, encouraged persons at risk for HIV infection to determine their HIV status rather than discouraging testing, as they had previously. In June 1997 the Gay Men's Health Crisis Center opened its own testing center.

Another controversy surrounding testing concerns reporting HIV-positive patients by name. Every state is required to report AIDS cases. As of December 2000, 34 states, Guam, and the Virgin Islands had implemented HIV case surveillance using the same confidential system for name-based case reporting for both HIV infection and AIDS. (See Table 9.1 for a list of states and territories with confidential HIV infection reporting.)

Two states conducted pediatric surveillance only (Connecticut and Oregon). The state of Washington has implemented HIV reporting by patient name to enable public health follow-up; after services and referrals are offered, names are converted into codes. In June 2000 New York, a state with high rates of HIV infection prevalence, instituted name reporting and partner notification legislation. In addition, at least six states (California, Illinois, Maine, Maryland, Massachusetts, and Pennsylvania) and Puerto Rico are reporting cases of HIV infection using a coded identifier rather than patient name. In most other states, HIV case reporting was under consideration or laws, rules, or regulations enabling HIV surveillance were expected to be implemented during 2002.

Critics, including the American Civil Liberties Union (ACLU), assail name-reporting as an invasion of privacy that carries social and economic risks. They claim that any benefit that would result from reporting names could not override the negative consequences (ostracism and loss of job and insurance, for instance) of being classified as

TABLE 9.1

States with confidential HIV infection reporting, through December 2000

Area of residence
(Date HIV reporting initiated)

Alabama (Jan. 1988)
Alaska (Feb. 1999)
Arizona (Jan. 1987)
Arkansas (July 1989)
Colorado (Nov. 1985)
Connecticut (July 1992)[2]
Florida (July 1997)
Idaho (June 1986)
Indiana (July 1988)
Iowa (July 1998)
Kansas (July 1999)
Louisiana (Feb. 1993)
Michigan (April 1992)
Minnesota (Oct. 1985)
Mississippi (Aug. 1988)
Missouri (Oct. 1987)
Nebraska (Sept. 1995)
Nevada (Feb. 1992)
New Jersey (Jan. 1992)
New Mexico (Jan. 1998)
North Carolina (Feb. 1990)
North Dakota (Jan. 1988)
Ohio (June 1990)
Oklahoma (June 1988)
Oregon (Sept. 1988)[2]
South Carolina (Feb. 1986)
South Dakota (Jan. 1988)
Tennessee (Jan. 1992)
Texas (Jan. 1999)[2]
Utah (April 1989)
Virginia (July 1989)
West Virginia (Jan. 1989)
Wisconsin (Nov. 1985)
Wyoming (June 1989)

U.S. dependencies, possessions, and associated nations

Guam (March 2000)
Virgin Islands, U.S (Dec. 1998)

[1]Includes only persons reported with HIV infection who have not developed AIDS.
[2]Connecticut has confidential HIV infection reporting for pediatric cases only; Oregon has confidential HIV infection reporting for children less than 6 years old. Texas reported only pediatric HIV infection cases from February 1994 until January 1999.

SOURCE: "Table 3. HIV infection cases by area and age group, reported through December 2000, from areas with confidential HIV infection reporting," in *HIV/AIDS Surveillance Report*, vol.12, no. 2, Centers for Disease Control and Prevention, Atlanta, GA, 2000

check the accuracy of testing labs, Katz states that not using name reporting "...essentially leaves us with is a big batch of nothing. We can tell how many positive tests have been reported, but I can't tell you how many human beings that represents."

Demographic data are used in states that do not require name reporting. During 1998 the Centers for Disease Control and Prevention (CDC) funded projects in Texas and Maryland that incorporated unique identifiers (the last four digits of the Social Security number, birth date, sex, and race), instead of names, for those tested. While the name-reporting debate continues, there is widespread agreement that testing is most effective if followed by counseling that completely explains the results and their consequences.

Counseling and Testing

Counseling and testing are important components of state and local HIV-prevention programs. Testing at publicly funded centers is free or costs only a nominal amount, while testing through a private physician can cost more than $200. In 2001 the CDC released a summary of the results of the *2000 Behavioral Risk Factor Surveillance System (BRFSS)* survey that has been conducted annually since 1991. Among its many objectives, the *BRFSS* survey evaluated differences in rates of testing and the receipt of HIV counseling and testing by state. Persons between the ages of 18 and 65 in 49 states and the District of Columbia responded to the telephone survey.

A median (half the states had more; half had less) of 45.7 percent of respondents reported having at least one HIV-antibody test; in 1998, a median of 40 percent of respondents had been tested for HIV. The 2000 survey found the proportions of those who had been tested for reasons other than donating blood ranged from a low of 35 percent in Minnesota to a high of 65.3 percent in the District of Columbia. Of those who had been tested for HIV, a median of 86.4 percent of persons reported receiving the results of their last HIV test; less than one-third of those tested (the median was 32.3 percent) received post-HIV test counseling.

Contact Tracing or Partner Notification

A by-product of testing is contact tracing, or partner notification. When individuals test positive for HIV, health officials ask them to provide, with the promise of anonymity, the names of those with whom they have had sexual contact or shared needles. The CDC asks counselors to inform contacts if the patient is reluctant to do so. The CDC strongly endorses contact-tracing programs, but results have varied. States struggling under the strain of numerous HIV/AIDS cases continue to support programs that encourage the infected persons to notify partners on their own. Contact-tracing programs in states with

infected. They add that name-reporting discourages those at risk for HIV from coming forward to seek testing and timely treatment.

The American Medical Association (AMA) and other advocates for reporting patients by name claim that it is essential for contact tracing, or partner notification, so that others who may have been infected will obtain treatment and other services. In Iowa, before name-reporting legislation had been adopted, John Katz, STD/HIV program manager for the state's Department of Public Health, claimed that it is virtually impossible to determine trends without name reporting. Because some patients have repeat tests, and because some tests are performed to

fewer HIV/AIDS cases are more likely to contact partners. Many patients who have HIV or AIDS fear that the promises of confidentiality will be broken; others fear retribution from those they may have infected.

More and more, states are trying to expand contact-tracing programs of health departments that notify sexual partners exposed to the virus. As an example, since 1995, health department counselors in Missouri's partner notification system have received additional training in teaching skills to reduce risky behavior. CDC-funded demonstration projects such as the San Francisco Bay Area Partner Assistance, Information, and Referral Services (PAIRS), which began in 1998, are trying to determine whether aggressive, confidential partner notification will prove to be an effective HIV prevention measure.

Home Testing

Home HIV tests were developed in the mid-1980s, but were opposed by the Food and Drug Administration (FDA) and some HIV/AIDS organizations and health care agencies. The FDA was concerned about telephone counseling for those who tested positive, the accuracy of the tests, and confidentiality. In 1996 the FDA reversed its position, deciding that despite its limitations, the benefits of home testing outweighed the risks.

The CDC claims that significant numbers of people have acquired HIV but do not know it. Many, say public health officials, are afraid of getting tested at a physician's office or public clinic because of the associated stigma. Some drug companies suggest that an HIV-antibody test that can be performed at home may be the only way some of these people will learn their HIV status, and argue that more people will then take steps to get treatment and prevent spreading the infection.

Some home tests use saliva, which does not require a needle stick, and others use blood samples. When blood is tested, the patient draws a few drops of blood from a fingertip, places it on filter paper, and mails the paper to a company laboratory, which performs the standard HIV assay. If the results are positive, a confirmation test is performed. An HIV test kit called Home Access Express HIV-1 Test System, manufactured by Home Access Health, was the only HIV home test kit approved by the FDA as of November 2001. Three days after the Home Access Express test kit is received by Home Access Health, results and counseling are available by calling a 24-hour toll-free number and giving an identification code. Home Access claims a greater than 99.9 percent accuracy rate.

Critics of home testing say that news of HIV infection is not as easy to accept as the results of other in-home tests, such as those for pregnancy and cholesterol. They claim that most people cannot properly prepare them-selves for the news that they have a life-threatening disease. They advocate expansion of current testing sites to include mobile vans, sports clubs, and other places that are not exclusively associated with HIV testing, but where in-person counseling could be provided.

Military Practices

The Department of Defense (DOD) regularly screens all members of the armed services, and those seeking to join, for HIV. Annual HIV testing is required of all personnel on active duty as well as all members of the reserves and National Guard. In 1995, after two months of debate on Capitol Hill, federal legislators scrapped a discharge provision that would have forced the DOD to dismiss members of the military within six months of testing positive for HIV. Along with HIV infection, a number of chronic conditions, including cancer, asthma, diabetes, heart disease, or complications of pregnancy, place troops on limited assignment, precluding them from overseas service or combat.

Debating the merits of permitting HIV-infected personnel to remain in the military, then representative Robert K. Dornan, a California Republican, argued that HIV-infected troops constituted a threat to military readiness. He explained that, because of the provision limiting the chronically ill to limited duty, they cannot serve overseas and must return to the U.S. during a time of cutbacks in defense resources. He added that the military could not afford to keep HIV-infected personnel if they were unable to perform all duties.

Responding to Dornan's plea to oust HIV-infected personnel, Frederick F.Y. Pang, assistant defense secretary for force management policy, said discharging was unnecessary and would not improve military readiness. Pang wrote that if HIV-infected military personnel could perform required duties there was no reason to separate them from others or remove them from the armed forces. Dornan tried to pass a legislative provision (part of the proposed 1997 DOD Authorization) that would discharge all HIV-positive military and would cut off benefits to dependents. However, the House and Senate voted 399–25 to overturn the discharge law, which had been part of the 1996 DOD authorization.

Currently, the DOD screens all new recruits and students entering the service academies and those in the college Reserve Officers' Training Corps (ROTC) program. Those who test positive for HIV are not permitted into military service. The State Department, Foreign Service, Peace Corps, and Job Corps also routinely test employees.

Pregnant Women and Newborns

The issue of testing newborns has placed the rights of mothers at odds with those of their newborns. States have kept HIV test results anonymous to preserve a mother's right to privacy. Civil libertarians and some groups that represent women, gays, and lesbians support anonymous testing, claiming that attaching names to test results would start governments down the "slippery slope" of mandatory testing of adults. They also raise further privacy concerns, contending that once names are known, there is no guarantee they will not fall into the hands of employers, insurance companies, and others who might discriminate on the basis of HIV status.

On the other hand, proponents of disclosure claim newborns that test HIV-positive could be denied adequate medical care because their parents are unaware of their status. Approximately 75 percent of babies who test positive for HIV immediately after birth do not actually develop the disease. If their mothers breast-feed, however, the babies may contract the infection from their mother's milk.

In May 1996 the U.S. House and Senate passed bills that would cut off federal money for HIV/AIDS treatment to states that fail to comply with the new disclosure requirements. President Clinton signed the Ryan White CARE Act Amendment (PL 104-146) requiring mandatory testing of newborns if too few pregnant women agree to voluntary testing. States must now test all newborns for HIV and notify parents of the results. In June 1996 New York became the first state to mandate that health officials tell parents the results of HIV tests that the state routinely performs on all newborns. Before June 1996 parents in New York did not receive results unless they requested them, as is still the case in most states.

Health Care Workers and Patients

There has been a continuing debate over whether health care workers, who, many believe, have an obligation to inform their patients about their own HIV status, should be required to be tested. Some fear that mandatory testing of health care workers could eventually lead to mandatory testing of patients. In 1998 only patients who exhibited or claimed risk-taking behaviors, or requested an HIV test, were tested for HIV. In today's medical setting, however, all patients are treated as potentially infectious, and treatment personnel are required to wear protective gloves and, for some invasive medical procedures, goggles and masks. These safety measures are known as "universal precautions."

Prisoners

The question of screening inmates for HIV antibodies has been even more controversial than screening persons in the general population. Prison officials feel pressure from lawmakers, city and county officials, correctional officers, and even inmates to perform mandatory screening of all inmates and to make their HIV status known. Testing prisoners raises the issue of spending resources for screening instead of educational materials. A number of prison systems engage in blind, anonymous prevalence studies where only overall results are made known and individual inmates are not told the test results. The majority of prison systems offer HIV testing for those who request it. (See Chapter 4, Table 4.7 for state guidelines.)

PREVENTION

Critics Fault Programs' Focus and Funding

The objective of HIV prevention programs is to reduce the number of new cases to as close to zero as possible. All prevention efforts are based on the belief that individuals can be educated in a way that will lead to a change in behavior, which will help bring an end to the spread of HIV/AIDS. However, many AIDS advocacy groups have long been critical of the ways the CDC has communicated the message. In 1987 CDC officials decided to emphasize the universality of AIDS, instead of focusing its efforts on those most at risk—men who have sex with men and intravenous drug users (IDUs). This, according to AIDS advocates, misdirected the spending of available prevention dollars. Today, although the number of infected people outside of those groups is growing, HIV/AIDS is still largely a threat to MSM, drug addicts, their partners, and their children. Most women with HIV/AIDS are drug users or sex partners of drug users.

This emphasis on the "anyone can get HIV" concept, critics claim, has diverted funds from the target populations with the greatest need for preventive health education. In 1995 the federal AIDS-prevention budget allocated no funds for programs aimed at MSM or for needle exchange programs. The CDC's 1996, $584 million AIDS prevention budget went largely to programs to help fight the disease among heterosexual women, college students, and others who face a relatively low risk of HIV infection. Through 1998 and 1999 funding from the Ryan White CARE Act served African Americans, Hispanics, and women in higher proportions than their representation in the AIDS population.

Hoping to change the way funds are appropriated, Ron Stall, associate professor of epidemiology at the University of California at San Francisco, argues that the AIDS epidemic cannot be stopped unless the prevention budget is spent where it can make the most difference— by targeting high-risk groups.

Dr. Helene Gayle, who heads AIDS prevention at the CDC, defends the agency's funding. "One should not underestimate the fear and confusion this disease caused early on," she says, referring to the 1987 decision. Dr. Gayle explains that the political and social forces at work at that time made it nearly impossible for the CDC to focus on those most at risk.

Those forces included attitudes concerning the morals of those with HIV and unlikely public support for funding

HIV/AIDS prevention programs directed solely towards MSM and drug users. According to Paula Van Ness, who worked at the CDC after managing an HIV/AIDS prevention program in Los Angeles, CDC officials decided to adopt an exaggerated heterosexual-risk policy, rather than jeopardize their prevention funding. They took this action because they believed that fighting HIV/AIDS was everyone's responsibility, even if everyone was not equally at risk. Those forces, says Dr. Gayle, still predominate, making it difficult for the government to change directions.

CDC Prevention Activities

The CDC believes its role is to prevent HIV infection and to reduce the illnesses and deaths that result from HIV infection by working with communities and other partners. The agency's efforts focus on:

- Monitoring the epidemic.
- Improving public understanding of the HIV epidemic.
- Preventing risk behaviors among students.
- Preventing and reducing behaviors and practices that transmit HIV.
- Increasing individual knowledge of HIV status and improving referral to appropriate prevention and treatment services.

The CDC stresses cooperation with, and provision of financial assistance and technical support to, state and local health and education agencies, national and local minority organizations, community-based organizations, schools and colleges, business and labor, and religious organizations. The CDC distributes almost 75 percent of its HIV prevention funds through grants and contracts, primarily to state and local health and education agencies.

EDUCATING YOUTH

By the end of 2000 more than 128,000 Americans between the ages of 20 and 29 had been diagnosed with AIDS. With an average incubation period of 10 years, it is likely that most of these young people were infected while they were teenagers. As some people begin having sexual relationships and using illegal drugs at earlier ages, many fear the number of HIV-positive young people will grow.

Most states offer prevention programs for students in public schools. According to a 1996 joint report prepared by the White House Office of National AIDS Policy, the National AIDS Fund, and the Until There's A Cure Foundation, however, HIV is hitting runaway and out-of-school youth hardest. These two groups are particularly difficult to reach with prevention information. Many homeless shelters and local health departments employ roving counselors who seek out these young people to offer prevention information and direct them to health and social service agencies.

Sexual Health Education

In 1997 the Joint United Nations Programme on HIV/AIDS (UNAIDS) reported that sex education for children and young people furthers safer sexual practices and does not increase sexual activity. UNAIDS based its findings on a review of 68 reports on sexual health education from France, Mexico, Switzerland, Thailand, the United Kingdom, and the United States, as well as from several Nordic countries.

The review focused on research on the behavioral impact of HIV/AIDS and sexual health education on young people. They compared the behavior of youths who received the education with those who did not. Some of the indicators included adolescent pregnancy rates, sexually transmitted disease (STD) infection rates, and self-reported sexual activity. The review concluded:

- Education about sexual health and/or HIV does not encourage more sexual activity.
- High-quality programs help delay first intercourse and protect sexually active youth from STDs, including HIV, and from pregnancy.
- Responsible and safe behavior can be learned.
- Sexual health education is best started before sexual activity begins.

Many education programs offer students sufficient information about STDs and HIV/AIDS, but only high-quality education affects behavior. The UNAIDS review concluded that effective education programs should include:

- Focused curricula, clear statements about behavioral goals, a clear picture of the risks of unprotected sex and ways to avoid it.
- Teaching and practice in communication and negotiation skills.
- Openness in communicating about sex.
- Theories stressing the social nature of learning.

Some people do not agree that information about sexual decisions should be offered in public schools, preferring that parents instill their own values in their children. However, others point out that some parents never talk to their children about sex and drugs, and school may be the only place a child can get reliable information. According to the National Conference of State Legislatures, 40 states, the District of Columbia, Puerto Rico, and the Virgin Islands require HIV/AIDS prevention education. Though laws vary from state to state, and some allow local school districts to decide on curriculum, many of these states have one or more mandates determining the material that may be taught in the programs. The mandates range from requiring age-appropriate materials to teaching comprehensive sexuality education programs (advocating contraceptive and condom use) to programs in which abstinence from pre-marital sex is presented as the only 100 percent effective means of preventing HIV/AIDS.

In 1996 the enactment of a federal entitlement program provided $50 million per year for five years (beginning in 1998) to be given in block grants to states that adhere to abstinence-only-until-marriage education programs. These programs prohibit discussion of condoms to prevent pregnancy or HIV/AIDS. Since then, another $50 million was allocated in competitive grants to states with these programs. According to some estimates, funding for these programs has increased nearly 3,000 percent since 1996.

Proponents of the abstinence-only programs state that the programs change attitudes about casual sex, reducing both teen pregnancies and rates of STDs. They also maintain that teaching students about contraceptive and condom use condones, or even encourages, unsafe sexual behavior. Critics of these programs argue that there is no reliable evidence that abstinence-only programs are effective. In addition, they contend that for the over 5 out of 10 teens from ages 15 to 19 who do choose to have sex, lack of knowledge about contraceptive and condom use will only result in continued teen pregnancies and HIV infections.

CONDOM USE

In 1993 the CDC released the pamphlet "Facts About Condoms and Their Use in Preventing HIV Infection and Other STDs" (Washington, D.C.). The CDC maintains that proper and consistent use of latex condoms when engaging in vaginal, anal, or oral sexual activity can reduce the risk of acquiring or transmitting STDs, including HIV. The publication stresses that studies provide compelling evidence that latex condoms are highly effective in protecting against HIV infection when used properly for every act of intercourse. It warns, however, that several studies have shown that condoms are not 100 percent effective. Breakage occurs in almost two percent of usage, usually due to the use of oil-based lubricants, exposure to heat or sunlight, or tearing by teeth or fingernails. (In 2001 latex condom use was still considered a highly effective method of preventing the transmission of HIV and other STDs.)

Other Forms of Protection

In 1993 the FDA approved Reality, a female condom that serves as a mechanical barrier to viruses. The condom is designed for women to protect themselves from STDs, including HIV. It is made of polyurethane (a resin made of two different compounds used in elastic fibers, cushions, and various molded products) and is unlikely to rip or tear. The condom is prelubricated, and is intended for use during only one sex act.

The role of spermicides in preventing HIV infection is uncertain. Condoms lubricated with spermicides are no more likely to be effective than condoms used with other water-based lubricants.

The CDC emphasizes that the transmission of STDs, including HIV infection, is preventable when an individual uses responsible prevention strategies. Abstinence is the most effective prevention strategy when it is practiced consistently. All other prevention strategies must be used correctly and consistently for them to be highly effective.

IMPROVING PREVENTION SERVICES

In March 2000 community planners, health educators and program directors met at the Community Planning Leadership Summit for HIV Prevention in Los Angeles, California, to share some of the most successful prevention and health education strategies from across the United States. By sharing these new and noteworthy "best practices," state health departments and local community planning groups were able to learn useful and proven approaches they could incorporate in their own programs.

The CDC reviewed the HIV prevention programs and compiled descriptions of them in a publication called *Bright Ideas 2000*. The publication was so well received that another edition, *Bright Ideas 2001: Innovative or Promising Practices in HIV Prevention and HIV Prevention Community Planning, Second Edition* followed, profiling additional programs from several jurisdictions that had not been represented in the previous edition.

Bright Ideas 2001 programs used innovative approaches to reach their target audiences, from an Alabama program that trained high school students to serve as peer group facilitators and counselors to an Iowa strategy to get members to arrive on time for meetings—latecomers were required to sing a song, tell a joke, or dance for the assembled group. A Louisiana program sought to improve its organizational ability to set priorities by using coded maps of STD rates, and in Maine a Web site helped people gain online access to HIV prevention information.

During 2000 the CDC also published the results of a study conducted by its Program Evaluation Research Branch (PERB). The PERB study tried to determine which factors help or hinder the efforts of community-based organizations (CBOs) that serve people at risk of acquiring or transmitting HIV. Using one-on-one and group interviews, PERB looked at 26 community-based organizations that varied in terms of target audience, geographic location, and type of services offered.

The PERB study found that some characteristics of the community such as support from city and local health departments, well-organized target populations, strong, supportive families and faith organizations, and well-established social networks were associated with the success of the CBOs in reaching their target audiences.

TABLE 9.2

Examples of factors that help and hinder community-based organizations to reach their target populations and deliver interventions

	Factors that Help	Factors that Hinder
Structural/ External	Supportive city and health department Well organized target population	Police harassment Limitations on the accessability of syringes Policies that prevent condom distribution Poverty Racism, sexism, drug phobia, homophobia
Cultural Norms	Strong role of families Active faith communities	Distrust of social service providers Ashamed to talk about sexuality
Client Factors	Well established social networks	High rates of drug use, poverty, unemployment, mental health issues, STDs, teen pregnancy, domestic violence, etc. Transient nature of clients Denial/clients tired of hearing about AIDS
Organizational	Long history in the community Credibility Clear mission/strong identity "One stop shopping:" multi-services	Overly bureaucratic management Insufficient support for line staff Insufficient infrastructure Abstinence/no condom distribution policy
Staff	Charismatic leader Flexible work environment Support for line staff Staff represent community Commitment / Work as a team	High turnover/vacancies Difficulty finding staff that represent target population Conflicts between staff Not enough money to pay staff
Program	Needs assessments Market research Realistic goals and objectives Incentives Meet clients "where they are at" "Infotainment"–combining education and entertainment Flexible implementation design	Unrealistic goals and objectives Inappropriate strategies for target population No meaningful integration of evaluation data

SOURCE: "Table 2. Examples of Factors that Help and hinder CBOs to Reach their Target Populations and Deliver Interventions," in *Learing from the Community What Community-Based Organizations Say About Factors that Affect HIV Prevention Programs,* Conwal Inc., Centers for Disease Control, September 2000

Characteristics of the CBOs themselves that helped them to reach their target groups included a long history in the community; a strong, clear mission and identity; and a charismatic leader (one easily able to gain the trust and devotion of the group). Effective CBOs also established realistic goals and objectives, developed programs to meet clients "where they are at," and delivered information in an entertaining way. (See Table 9.2.)

Factors that hampered the effectiveness of the CBOs were high rates of poverty, racism, sexism, drug use and homophobia, teen pregnancy, and domestic violence, along with transient client populations. Policies that prevented condom distribution, not enough money to pay CBO staff, and limitations on the accessibility of syringes also prevented CBOs from reaching their target populations. (See Table 9.2.)

SYRINGE EXCHANGE PROGRAMS (SEPS)

In April 1998, after much debate, the Clinton administration decided not to lift a nine-year-old ban on federal financing for programs to distribute clean needles to drug addicts. This means that state and local governments that receive federal block grants for HIV/AIDS prevention are not permitted to use that money for needle exchange pro-

grams. Public health experts and advocates for people with HIV/AIDS criticized the decision. Later in 1998 Congress considered even more restrictive legislation that would ban indirect federal funding (such as funding for counseling, medical care, or funds dispersed by city or state) to needle exchange agencies. Regardless, in 2000 five U.S. health groups (including the American Medical Association and the American Pharmaceutical Association) spoke in favor of needle exchange programs, and advised state leaders to coordinate efforts to make clean needles easily available to intravenous drug users (IDUs).

Federal officials estimate that each day 33 people are infected with HIV as a result of intravenous drug use. This figure includes IDUs, their sexual partners, and their children. According to Surgeon General David Satcher, intravenous drug use is also responsible for most of the spread of HIV/AIDS, particularly among the poor and minorities. He said that 40 percent of all new HIV/AIDS infections in the United States result directly or indirectly from infection from contaminated needles. The figure among women and children is 75 percent.

The *Monthly Morbidity and Mortality Report,* in "Update: Syringe Exchange Programs—United States, 1998" (Vol. 47, No. 31, August 14, 1998), summarized a

TABLE 9.3

Syringe exchange statistics, 1998

Size	No. syringes exchanged per SEP	No. SEPs	Total no. syringes exchanged	% syringes exchanged
Small	<10,000	30	108,136	1%
Medium	10,000–55,000	26	778,701	4%
Large	55,001–499,999	39	6,398,409	33%
Very large	>500,000	12	12,112,281	62%
Total		**107**	**19,397,527**	**100%**

Note: SEP means syringe exchange program.

SOURCE: "Table 1. Number of syringe exchange programs (SEPs), number of syringes exchanged per SEP, total number of syringes, and percentage of total number of syringes, by program size category—United States, 1998," in "Update, Syringe Exchange Programs—United States, 1998," *Morbidity and Mortality Weekly Report,* vol. 50, no. 19, May 18, 2001

survey of U.S. syringe exchange program (SEP) activities during 1998. In October 1999 the Beth Israel Medical Center (BIMC) in New York City, together with the North American Syringe Exchange Network (NASEN), mailed questionnaires to the directors of 131 SEPs in the U.S. who were members of NASEN. (Previous surveys contacted 68 SEPs during 1994–1995, 101 in 1996, and 113 in 1997.) BIMC contacted the SEP directors and conducted telephone interviews based on the questionnaires. The directors responded to questions about the number of syringes exchanged during 1998, program operations, and services provided.

Of the 131 SEPs, 110 (84 percent) participated in the survey, but some SEPs asked that their data be reported only as aggregate. The SEPs operated in 81 cities in 31 states, the District of Columbia, and Puerto Rico. The greatest numbers of SEPs were located in four states: California (21), New York (14), Washington (12), and New Mexico (9). Nine cities had at least two SEPs.

In 1998, the 107 individually-reporting SEPs exchanged approximately 19.4 million syringes, up from the 1997 total of 17.5 million. The 12 largest SEPs (those that traded 500,000 or more syringes) exchanged approximately 10.3 million (62 percent of all replaced syringes). (See Table 9.3.)

In addition to exchanged syringes, most SEPs provided other public health and social services. Virtually all offered instruction in preventing sexual transmission of HIV and other sexually transmitted diseases (STDs); 98 percent provided male condoms and 73 percent distributed female condoms. Ninety-nine percent provided IDUs with alcohol pads, 90 percent offered bleach to use as disinfectant, and 95 percent referred clients to substance abuse treatment programs. Other on-site health care services provided by some SEPs included HIV counseling and testing (64 percent), tuberculosis skin testing (15 percent), STD screening (14 percent) and primary health care (19 percent).

Helping IDUs Saves Lives

The CDC, in "Changing Syringe Laws Is Part of Strategy to Help Stem HIV Spread" (*HIV/AIDS Prevention*, Atlanta, Georgia, December 1997), pointed out that drug users must have access to clean syringes and drug treatment as part of a complete HIV prevention plan. One way to make this happen is to change the drug paraphernalia laws so that clean needles and syringes are available to IDUs. However, many people believe that by doing so, the state is allowing drug use to take place, or even worse, condoning it.

The Public Health Service policy recommends that IDUs be counseled and encouraged to stop using and injecting drugs, if possible, through substance abuse treatment that includes relapse prevention. Failing this, however, drug users should follow various preventive plans that include:

- Never reusing or sharing syringes, water, or drug preparation equipment.

- Using only syringes obtained from a reliable source (e.g., pharmacies).

- Using a new, sterile syringe to prepare and inject drugs.

- Safely disposing of syringes after one use.

Despite social and economic obstacles to their success, SEPs have repeatedly demonstrated that they can assist to change the lives of IDUs. Research reported in *Public Health Reports* in "A Drug Abuse Treatment Success among Needle Exchange Participants" (Supplement 1, June 1998) found that 50 percent of clients referred for substance abuse treatment entered treatment and 76 percent completed 13 weeks of treatment. These findings were especially impressive in view of the programs' clientele—persons with more severe drug abuse, more HIV risk behaviors, and more participation in illegal activities than IDUs referred to treatment from other sites.

Legislation in Maine and Minnesota

A 1997 law in Maine (Maine Statute, Title 32, Ch. 117, Sect. 32, Para. 13787-A) permits anyone to legally possess 10 or fewer syringes. "Illegal possession" of syringes applies to anyone who knowingly owns or furnishes 11 or more syringes, except those who must self-inject prescription drugs (like insulin-dependent diabetics) and syringe exchange program (SEP) operators, who are not limited in the quantity of syringes they possess. The statute authorizes the state Bureau of Health to establish SEPs and set the rules that will govern them. SEPs must keep track of and dispose of syringes, they must have drug prevention education, and they are required to submit an annual report on the operation of their programs.

Legislation in Minnesota (Minnesota Statute Section 151 Para. 40) modified its drug paraphernalia law so that pharmacists are permitted to sell, and IDUs to buy, 10 or fewer syringes. The Commissioner of Health is now required to give pharmacists help with technical issues, such as proper disposal of used syringes and provision of materials needed to make the program work.

Legal Barriers to Federal Funding of Needle Exchange Programs

Regardless of the evidence from a number of sources that needle exchange programs are effective strategies for HIV transmission, the federal government, as well as most local and state governments, have not made them legal. They argue that illicit drug use should not be financed by taxpayers. Since 1988 Congress has passed at least six laws that contain provisions specifically prohibiting or restricting use of federal funds for needle exchange programs and activities. The Comprehensive Alcohol Abuse, Drug Abuse, and Mental Health Amendments Act of 1988 (PL 100-690) required states, as a condition for receiving block grant funds, to agree that funds would not be used "to carry out any programs of distributing sterile needles for hypodermic injection of an illegal drug or distributing bleach for the purpose of cleansing needles for such hypodermic injection."

CHAPTER 10
HIV AND AIDS WORLDWIDE

SCOPE OF THE PROBLEM

Besides the increasing world population, few factors have changed global demographics as inalterably as the pandemic (worldwide epidemic) of HIV/AIDS. For instance, United Nations officials have projected that sub-Saharan African countries will be 4 percent less populated in the year 2005 than they would have been without the losses attributable to AIDS. By 2025, according to information released in 1996 by the International Programs Center of the U.S. Census Bureau, the sub-Saharan population would have reached almost 1.3 billion without AIDS. A moderate spread of AIDS, however, could reduce that number by more than 100 million.

The HIV/AIDS pandemic is actually many separate epidemics, each with its own distinctive origin, shaped by specific geography and populations. Each epidemic involves different risk behaviors and practices, such as unprotected sex with multiple partners or sharing drug injection equipment. It is estimated that, in a half-dozen sub-Saharan African countries, the majority of the "high-risk" urban population—prostitutes and their customers and sexually transmitted disease patients—are HIV-positive. International authorities project that unless the rate of HIV/AIDS infection slows in 13 sub-Saharan countries, Brazil, and Haiti, childhood mortality rates could triple by the year 2010.

In 1997, approximately 30.6 million people were infected with HIV, and the pandemic was growing by 16,000 new infections per day. By the end of 2000 the Joint United Nations Programme on HIV/AIDS (UNAIDS) and the World Health Organization (WHO) estimated that approximately 36.1 million people worldwide were living with HIV. (See Figure 10.1.) During that year, 5.3 million people were newly infected with HIV (14,520 per day) and 3 million people died of AIDS. Approximately 2.2 million women were newly infected with HIV during 2000 (comprising 42 percent of all new HIV infections).

The AIDS epidemic had left behind a cumulative total of more than 12 million orphans by the end of 2000.

United Nations medical experts note that, before 1997, data coming from just a few countries in any particular area were used as models for other countries with comparable or fairly similar regional factors. As a result, for some countries the spread of HIV/AIDS was woefully underestimated. Starting in 1997, separate models constructed for each country replaced regional models, and the results are more accurate statistics and projections.

UNAIDS estimates that, in 2000, 3 million people worldwide died from AIDS, up from 2.3 million in 1997. Nearly half (1.3 million) of those deaths were women. In 2000, 500,000 children throughout the world died of AIDS, up from 460,000 in 1997. UNAIDS also estimates that, in 2000, 600,000 children under 15 were newly infected with HIV. Worldwide, 1.4 million children were living with HIV/AIDS in 2000. Part of the increase is attributable to better reporting, but much of it results from the uncontrolled spread of the disease.

WHO reports that over two-thirds (70 percent) of the world's HIV-infected population lives in sub-Saharan Africa; another 16 percent reside in South and Southeast Asia, and an additional 4 percent are in Latin America. (See Figure 10.1.) WHO reports that of the 5.3 million newly infected people in 2000, 3.8 million lived in sub-Saharan Africa, 780,000 lived in South and Southeast Asia, and 30,000 were in Western Europe. In 2000, there were 60,000 new infections in the Caribbean, more than the 45,000 in North America.

In order to understand the enormity and consequences of the AIDS pandemic worldwide, the focus should not be on the number of reported AIDS cases, but instead on the number of persons infected with HIV (the virus that causes AIDS), most of whom have not yet developed full-blown AIDS. The HIV incubation period, the interval

FIGURE 10.1

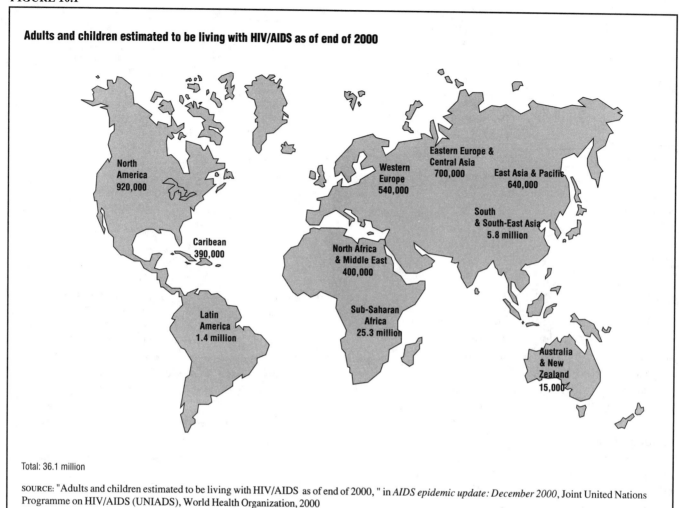

Adults and children estimated to be living with HIV/AIDS as of end of 2000

North America
920,000

Caribean
390,000

Latin America
1.4 million

Western Europe
540,000

Eastern Europe & Central Asia
700,000

East Asia & Pacific
640,000

South & South-East Asia
5.8 million

North Africa & Middle East
400,000

Sub-Saharan Africa
25.3 million

Australia & New Zealand
15,000

Total: 36.1 million

SOURCE: "Adults and children estimated to be living with HIV/AIDS as of end of 2000," in *AIDS epidemic update: December 2000*, Joint United Nations Programme on HIV/AIDS (UNIADS), World Health Organization, 2000

between the initial HIV infection and the development of AIDS, is estimated to be about 7–11 years.

Global Trends and Projections

Although public health activities have made impressive progress in eliminating and controlling many infectious diseases in the past 20 years, HIV/AIDS is not one of them, according to WHO. This is due to the constantly changing character and the complex role of factors that determine the progression from HIV infection to full-blown AIDS. In addition, medical treatments that can slow the progression of HIV infection are generally too expensive, and as a result inaccessible, for most people living in developing countries.

The World Bank projects that by 2020 AIDS will account for a large portion of deaths from infectious diseases in the developing world. Figure 10.2 shows projected deaths from HIV/AIDS as a percentage of deaths from infectious diseases in various parts of the world. In Latin America and the Caribbean, 74 percent of adults who die from an infectious disease will likely die from HIV/AIDS,

while in the Middle East and North Africa, only 18 percent of adults who die from an infectious disease will likely die from HIV/AIDS.

Figure 10.3 shows the percentage of adult deaths due to infectious diseases in 1990 and the forecasted percentage for 2020. In 1990, HIV/AIDS accounted for 9 percent of adult deaths due to infectious diseases; however, by 2020 HIV/AIDS is projected to account for 37 percent of adult deaths due to infectious diseases. The following observations describe the nature of the HIV/AIDS pandemic in 1998, which, without effective interventions, should develop in a similar manner through 2010:

• Most new adult HIV infections occurred in 15- to 24-year-olds.

• Three-fourths or more (75–85 percent) of HIV-positive adults worldwide were infected through unprotected sex. Heterosexual (men/women) intercourse accounted for more than 70 percent; and MSM (men who have sex with men) accounted for 5–10 percent.

FIGURE 10.2

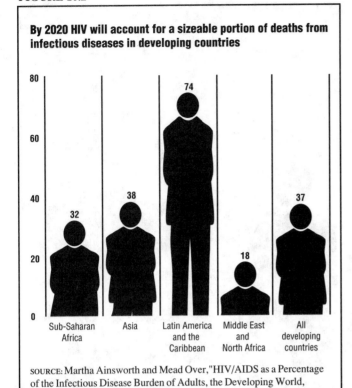

By 2020 HIV will account for a sizeable portion of deaths from infectious diseases in developing countries

SOURCE: Martha Ainsworth and Mead Over,"HIV/AIDS as a Percentage of the Infectious Disease Burden of Adults, the Developing World, 2020," in *Confronting AIDS: Public Priorities in a Global Epidemic*, The World Bank, Oxford University Press, 1998

- Transfusions of HIV-infected blood caused 3–5 percent of all global adult infections.

- Sharing HIV-infected injection equipment by drug users accounted for 5–10 percent worldwide.

- More than 90 percent of HIV-positive children throughout the world were infected by their mothers perinatally (before or during birth), or through breast-feeding. Approximately 30 percent of mother-to-child transmission took place through breastfeeding.

Effect of AIDS on Birth and Death Rates

Life expectancy at birth is an important measure for comparing death rates within and between countries over time. In some countries hardest hit by AIDS, the number of years one may expect to live has returned to the levels of the 1960s. Other countries now have levels equivalent to those of 10 years ago, and child survival rates are slipping as well. Even in countries with a somewhat lower prevalence of HIV infection, AIDS accounts for 80 percent of deaths of persons between 25 and 34 years of age.

In the sub-Saharan African nation of Zimbabwe, one of the countries hardest hit by the AIDS pandemic, life expectancy is only 42 years—22 years less than it would be if not for the impact of AIDS. In Harare, the capital of Zimbabwe, deaths among children 5 years or younger rose from 8 per 1,000 in 1988 to 20 per 1,000 in 1996. In

FIGURE 10.3

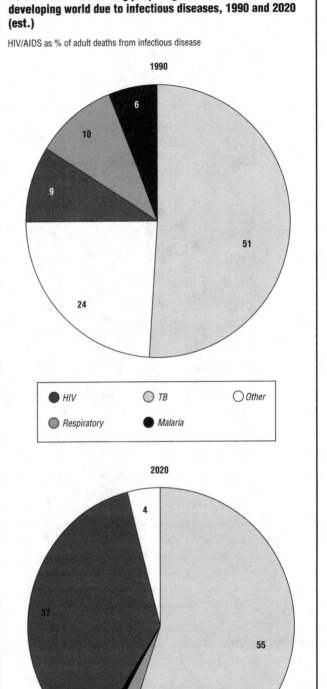

Percent of deaths among people ages 15 to 59 in the developing world due to infectious diseases, 1990 and 2020 (est.)

HIV/AIDS as % of adult deaths from infectious disease

1990

1990 legend: HIV, TB, Other, Respiratory, Malaria

2020

SOURCE: Martha Ainsworth and Mead Over,"Breakdown of Deaths from Infectious Diseases, the Developing World, by Disease Category, 1990 and 2020 (percent)" in *Confronting AIDS: Public Priorities in a Global Epidemic*, The World Bank, Oxford University Press, 1997

FIGURE 10.4

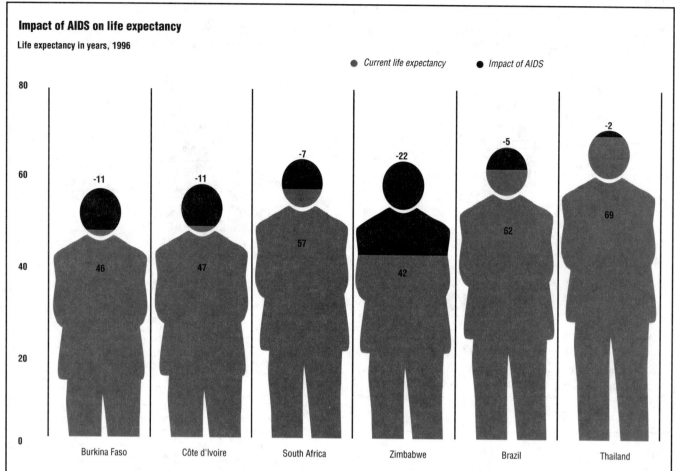

Impact of AIDS on life expectancy

Life expectancy in years, 1996

● *Current life expectancy* ● *Impact of AIDS*

SOURCE: Martha Ainsworth and Mead Over,"The Current Impact of AIDS on Life Expectancy, Six Selected Countries, 1996," in *Confronting AIDS: Public Priorities in a Global Epidemic*, The World Bank, Oxford University Press, 1998

East Africa, where 10 percent of the rural population has HIV, adult mortality has more than doubled. In southern Africa life expectancy between 2005–2010 is expected to drop to 45 years (from 59 years in the early 1990s), largely as a result of AIDS. In Brazil, a South American country, one may expect a life span of 62 years, 5 years shorter than a decade ago. In the Asian country of Thailand, where strong prevention programs are in place, the life span is 69 years, just 2 years shorter than a decade ago. (See Figure 10.4.)

Because HIV/AIDS epidemics differ considerably from country to country, most current mortality estimates, especially in developing countries, do not accurately reflect the impact of AIDS-related mortality. The HIV/AIDS epidemic is changing the course of demographic events in developing countries where the impact has been particularly severe.

WORLDWIDE AIDS DEATHS. The United Nations estimates that, from the beginning of the epidemic to the end of 2000, 21.8 million people had died from HIV/AIDS-related causes worldwide. Deaths in 2000 alone account-

ed for 14 percent of all deaths attributed to HIV/AIDS since the start of the epidemic. Sub-Saharan Africa was hit hardest; more than 17 million (almost 80 percent) of all AIDS-related deaths were in that area. In Southeast Asia, nearly a half-million people died of AIDS during 2000, for a total of just under 1.6 million. North American deaths from AIDS totaled 470,000 and Caribbean countries accounted for 192,000 AIDS deaths. Latin America suffered 570,000 AIDS deaths, while 217,000 people died of AIDS in Western Europe.

PATTERNS OF INFECTION

Globally, HIV/AIDS is primarily a sexually transmitted disease (STD), transmitted through unprotected sexual intercourse between men and women or men who have sex with men (MSM). Like some other STDs, HIV infection can also be spread through blood, blood products, donated organs, or semen, and perinatally from a woman to her unborn child. More than 75 percent of worldwide cumulative HIV infections in adults are estimated to have been transmitted through heterosexual intercourse, although the relative proportion of infections resulting from heterosexual contact as opposed to MSM varies greatly in different parts of the world.

HIV-1 and HIV-2

Two types of HIV have been recognized and identified: HIV-1, the predominant worldwide virus, and HIV-2. HIV-1 and HIV-2 show an extraordinary difference in global distribution. In North and South America, HIV-1 has reached epidemic proportions among certain risk groups, primarily through unprotected MSM contact and intravenous drug use (IDU). Some African and Asian countries have also experienced extensive heterosexual transmission of HIV-1. HIV-2 has spread among heterosexual populations in West Africa.

DIFFERENCES IN EPIDEMIOLOGY, INCIDENCE, AND TRANSMISSION. The epidemiological characteristics (the factors, such as distribution and incidence, that determine the presence, extent, or absence of a disease) of HIV-2 are different from HIV-1, and the international spread of HIV-2 is quite limited. In "Epidemiology and Transmission of HIV-2: Why There Is No HIV-2 Pandemic" (*Journal of the American Medical Association*, Vol. 270, No. 17, 1993), Dr. Kevin DeCock and colleagues reported that in the early course of infection, persons with HIV-2 are less infectious than those with HIV-1. This is due to the low levels of the virus isolated from the blood of immunodeficient persons with HIV-2. As time passes and an individual's immunodeficiency progresses, HIV-2 probably becomes more infectious, but this more infectious period is relatively shorter than for HIV-1 and tends to occur in older individuals.

Several studies have provided reasonable evidence that HIV-2 is not frequently transmitted from mother to child. While the mechanics of perinatal transmission are not completely understood, advanced immunodeficiency of the mother is certainly a risk factor. Low levels of the virus are not sufficient to transmit to the baby and, as mentioned above, higher levels of virus infection in women past childbearing years may explain why perinatal transmission is less frequent. This is the most likely explanation for the observation that HIV-2 infection is so rare in children.

Interactions and HIV Transmission

One of the major concerns of public health officials worldwide is the possible interaction between HIV and other infections. The same risky behaviors that expose individuals to potential HIV infection also expose them to other sexually transmitted diseases (STDs) such as gonorrhea, syphilis, and chancroid (a genital ulcer). Considerable data suggests that STDs, particularly herpes simplex, chancroid, and syphilis (which cause ulcerative lesions) promote the transmission of HIV.

TUBERCULOSIS. HIV infection is recognized as the strongest known risk factor for the development of active tuberculosis (TB), since people with latent TB infection are more apt to develop the disease once their immune system has been compromised by HIV. Latent TB infection is believed to be present in about 30–50 percent of adults in most developing countries. Persons with latent TB have positive tuberculosis skin tests (PPD) but are not sick with tuberculosis—they have been infected with *Mycobacterium tuberculosis* at some point in their lives but have not developed active TB.

As much as 8 percent of persons infected with both latent TB and HIV are expected to develop active TB each year. WHO estimates that at least four million adults worldwide, primarily in sub-Saharan Africa, Latin America, and Asia, have been infected with both HIV and *Mycobacterium tuberculosis*. Not only are persons who test tuberculin-positive and are also infected with HIV more likely to develop TB, but they also are likely to develop TB more rapidly than persons without HIV infection. An even more disastrous consequence is that half of all dually infected people will develop contagious TB, which they could then spread to any susceptible individual, even those not infected with HIV. Currently TB kills about two million people annually in developing countries, a figure that has grown dramatically since the HIV/AIDS epidemic has swept through many countries. The number of cases will continue to grow.

GEOGRAPHIC DIFFERENCES. In North America and Western Europe during the 1980s and early 1990s, HIV was transmitted predominantly through unprotected sexual intercourse among men (MSM) and through intravenous drug use (IDU) with contaminated needles. During the late-1990s heterosexual intercourse and IDU became the prevailing modes of HIV transmission in North America and Europe.

In sub-Saharan Africa the overwhelming mode of transmission has been heterosexual intercourse. In that part of the world, transmission through MSM contact or through IDU is slight. Because many women have been infected, rates of perinatal transmission are increasing. In 2000, 90 percent of HIV-positive babies born worldwide were in sub-Saharan Africa.

The rates of MSM transmission in Latin America are similar to those of Europe and the United States, but IDU is less frequent, while heterosexual transmission is considerably higher. In South and Southeast Asia, the rapid increase of HIV can be traced to shared contaminated injection equipment and heterosexual intercourse.

In other areas, such as East Asia and the Pacific region, the predominant modes of transmission are not as clearly defined because of the relatively recent (late-1980s) spread of HIV in these areas. While the infection rate has peaked in other parts of the world, it is escalating in Asia, mainly from heterosexual intercourse through prostitution. By the end of 2000 South and Southeast Asia had nearly 6.6 million adults and children living with HIV/AIDS; 770,000 adults and children were infected with HIV/AIDS in East Asia and the Pacific region.

AFRICA

Rural Africa Catching Up

In 1976, Dr. Nzila Nzilambi, of the Mama Yemo Hospital in Kinshasa, Zaire, tested for HIV, the virus that causes AIDS, in blood samples taken from residents of a remote province of Zaire. Five of the more than 650 samples—almost 1 percent—tested positive for HIV. Researchers returned in 1985 and sampled 389 people. Three were infected, the same proportion as nine years earlier.

At one time, HIV infection apparently existed at stable levels in rural regions of Africa. In urban areas, however, the virus spread through increased sexual activity and the relaxing of traditional tribal values. As more poor rural workers left their villages to search for jobs, the epidemic spread. Able-bodied workers often cannot bring their families with them when they leave their homes to seek work; and many take new sexual partners in the cities where they work. These workers return to their villages, bringing HIV and other STDs with them.

Unparalleled Infection Rates

By 1998 more than 7 percent of persons between the ages of 15 and 49 in sub-Saharan Africa were infected with HIV. This region is the hardest-hit area in the world. In early 1997 the South African government estimated that 2.4 million South Africans were living with HIV. The most recent *Report on the Global HIV/AIDS Epidemic* (prepared by the Joint United Nations Programme on HIV/AIDS and the World Health Organization, Geneva, June 2000) found a wide range of national prevalence rates (the number of cases of the disease present in a specified population at a given time) of HIV infection among adults. Some West African countries reported less than 2 percent. Others, in the southern portion of the continent, saw rates as high as 20 percent. The countries of Botswana and Zimbabwe have the highest rates of HIV infection. In those countries, as many as 25 percent of adults are infected. The disease has spread more rapidly in sub-Saharan Africa than in any other region of the world.

SEVERAL MODES OF TRANSMISSION. Because heterosexual transmission is the predominant mode of transmission in Africa, men and women appear to be almost equally infected—12–13 females per every 10 males. Commercial sex workers, or prostitutes, and their customers play a significant role in the spread of HIV in many countries. In many African cities the risk of contracting HIV infection approaches 50 percent. In some cities, infection is rampant, especially among sex workers in the lower socioeconomic class.

In the late 1990s four out of five HIV-positive women in the world lived in Africa, as did 87 percent of children who live with HIV. There are several reasons for this. The female childbearing population is larger in Africa than any other place, and African women generally have more children than women in other parts of the world. This means that one woman can pass the virus on to more children. Further, nearly all children in Africa are breastfed, and breastfeeding is responsible for more than one-third of mother-to-child transmissions of HIV. Although there are new drugs and drug combinations available to sharply reduce mother-to-child transmission, they are expensive and women in developing countries generally cannot afford them.

In response to routine screening of donated blood and the more careful use of blood for procedures such as transfusions, the role of transmission through HIV-infected blood has diminished considerably over the past several years, accounting for less than 10 percent of the total reported HIV infections. Ancient practices of ritual scarification and the use of improperly sterilized skin-piercing instruments (e.g., needles and syringes) account for a very small proportion of all HIV infections in sub-Saharan Africa.

PAYING THE PRICE FOR YEARS OF EVASION. Although their country had experienced the ravages of AIDS for at least a decade, Kenya's Parliament and Cabinet did not debate the issue publicly until 1993. Physicians diagnosed the first AIDS cases in 1984, but the government did not issue national statistics until 1986, when it announced one AIDS-related death. Although the nation's president and vice-president regularly warned the public in speeches to avoid infection, and national officials instructed district administrators, including local tribal chiefs, to encourage their people to practice safe sex and limit their partners, there had been no official statement.

The government's belated commitment to dealing with HIV/AIDS came too late for many Kenyans. By 2000, 2.1 million citizens had been infected with HIV; this represents nearly 15 percent of all sexually active adults. About 600 deaths per day in Kenya are attributable to AIDS, and by 2005 this number is projected to climb to 820 deaths per day. Moreover, the National AIDS/STD Control Programme (NASCP) estimates that more than 730,000 Kenyan children under the age of 15 have lost their mothers to AIDS. NASCP projects that this number will reach 1 million by 2005.

Kenya's reticence and seeming inability to deal with the epidemic came as a surprise to many observers. Kenya has endured an economic decline that many blame on corruption and the collapse of global commodity prices. Nonetheless Kenya is still one of Africa's wealthiest countries and has remained relatively stable since gaining its independence from Britain in 1963. Many observers thought that if any African country could cope with or even head off an HIV/AIDS epidemic, it would be Kenya.

However, Kenya chose to downplay the threat, lest it frighten away much-needed tourist dollars. Its neighbor Uganda, by contrast, began an aggressive campaign against the spread of HIV/AIDS in the mid-1980s, when it had the highest number of recorded HIV cases in Africa. With virtually every family touched by HIV/AIDS, much of the cultural, religious, and psychological stigma has disappeared in Uganda, where HIV infection rates now appear to be declining. In Kenya, on the other hand, many HIV-infected persons still mistakenly believed, many years after the epidemic first hit, that the absence of symptoms meant they were not infected.

Kenyan authorities have now developed a long-term strategy to deal with the epidemic that by 2010 will orphan more than 30 percent of Kenyan children under age 15. In 1997, Parliament adopted Sessional Paper No. 4. The law called for a vigorous campaign aimed at changing society's attitudes towards casual sex and proposing that anyone who intentionally infects another with HIV be found guilty of manslaughter.

Much of the HIV/AIDS epidemic in Kenya and other nations of East Africa can be attributed to the preponderance of wars and political upheaval. In addition, many prostitutes reside along long-haul truck routes linking Tanzanian and Kenyan ports to landlocked interior nations—Ethiopia, Uganda, Rwanda, Burundi, and the eastern part of Zaire. Recently, male and female adolescents between the ages of 15 and 19 have begun to frequent truck stops along the Trans-Africa Highway in Kenya. Teenagers in families that cannot adequately provide them with food and clothing trade sex for money and gifts.

International experts report that HIV in these areas is also prevalent among persons with higher-paying jobs, such as businessmen in Nairobi and Mombasa and truck drivers who frequent the roads between the eastern coast and the interior. It is not uncommon or socially unacceptable for a man of means to have a family as well as a couple of girlfriends. As in other parts of Africa, the big cities draw men from rural areas in search of work. Separated from their families for several months, many of these men turn to prostitutes and eventually contract HIV and carry it home to their villages. A considerable number of women in the cities who are abandoned or need additional income turn to prostitution to eke out a living.

"Wife inheritance" was once a socially useful tradition; now, it is a large contributor to the ever-increasing spread of HIV/AIDS. In western Kenya, when a woman is widowed, her former husband's family takes care of her and her children. For generations, a brother-in-law or male cousin took her in with his family. Initially, tradition

frowned on his having sexual relations with the inherited wife. Unfortunately, the inheritors began to ignore that restriction and had sex with the widow. If the widow's former husband had died of AIDS, she was likely to be infected and could pass the infection on to her inheritor, who would pass it on to his wife, causing the disease to multiply exponentially.

A report issued jointly by NASCP and the U.S.-based Family Health International, published in 1996 and released in 1997, warned that unless Kenya's government makes some changes quickly, HIV could destroy the country's economy. According to *AIDS in Kenya; Socioeconomic Impact and Policy Implications*, the total cost of AIDS to Kenya could reach 118 trillion Kenyan shillings (about $1.9 trillion American) by 2005.

UGANDA'S DECLINING HIV RATES. Scientists think that more than 20 years ago truck drivers first spread HIV in Uganda's Rakai district, which lies along a Victoria Lake trade route to the capital city of Kampala. Because commercial sex is widely available along the trade route, HIV quickly spread throughout Uganda and all of Africa. At one time, Uganda had the world's highest HIV infection rates. Today, Uganda is one of only two developing nations (Thailand is the other) where there is nationwide evidence of declining HIV rates due to strong prevention programs. According to the United Nations, Uganda reduced the prevalence of HIV infection by more than one-fourth, from almost 13 percent in 1994 to 8 percent in 1998.

Uganda was the first African country to respond strongly to its HIV/AIDS epidemic. The government began by gathering religious and traditional leaders along with representatives of other sectors of society, in an effort to reach agreement that the problem had to be confronted. Prevention efforts targeted specific populations or communities. For example, prevention programs that focused on delaying sexual relations and behaving in a safe manner were presented in schools. Community groups were formed to counsel and support those living with the virus. Condom use was heavily promoted.

Infection rates, particularly for the young, have begun to fall in both rural and urban surveillance sites. In 1989, 69 percent of 15- to 19-year-old males and 74 percent of 15- to 19-year-old females reported that they had had sexual intercourse. By 1995 those percentages had dropped to 44 percent among the young men and 54 percent among the young women. Young Ugandans seem to be postponing sexual initiation, seeking fewer sexual partners, and using condoms more.

EUROPE

Western Europe

While HIV in Europe is spread primarily through MSM contact, IDU is gaining as a mode of transmission.

In 1985 about 63 percent of AIDS cases among adult Europeans were due to MSM contact. By 1992, however, that proportion had dropped to 42 percent, while the proportion of European AIDS cases attributable to IDU jumped more than sevenfold, from 5 percent in 1985 to 36 percent in 1992.

According to the American Centers for Disease Control and Prevention (CDC), the reported number of AIDS cases stabilized in 1994 and 1995. In 1996, the number of AIDS cases reported throughout the European Union (EU) dropped about 10 percent. In 1997, CDC statistics indicated that the AIDS epidemic had declined sharply in Western Europe (39 percent); UNAIDS reported 30,000 new cases in Western Europe in 1997. Since the late 1990s, the decline appears to have leveled off; 30,000 new cases were reported in 2000 and 540,000 persons were estimated to be living with HIV/AIDS. The majority of HIV transmission in Spain and Italy was through IDU, while in France, Germany, and the United Kingdom, it was through MSM contact. Mother-to-child transmission rates were low due to the availability of antiretroviral drugs for pregnant women and safe alternatives to breast-feeding for HIV-infected mothers. UNAIDS estimates that fewer than 500 children under the age of 15 were infected with HIV in 2000.

SPAIN. Of all EU nations, Spain has the highest number of HIV/AIDS cases per capita. The first case of HIV was reported in Spain in 1981; by 1997 that number had grown to 46,600. Spain accounts for one-fourth of all HIV cases in Western Europe. (Italy and Portugal also have high rates of HIV/AIDS cases.)

Drug use in Spain began to increase during the 1970s and 1980s after the long Franco dictatorship ended. Dr. Isabel Noguer of the Health Ministry described this period as a time of heavy heroin use, with addicts sharing infected needles. In 1997 drug users still made up the highest risk group, while unprotected heterosexual relations was the next most common form of transmission. According to Spain's Health Ministry in 2000, 56 percent of HIV infections among men and 48 percent among women were attributable to IDU while heterosexual transmission was responsible for 22 percent of all cases (male and female).

Spain developed education and prevention programs, and the number of new cases began to level off in 1996. The Health Ministry gives more than $1 million in aid to 200 non-governmental groups annually. Condom sales in the mid-1990s were double the number in the 1980s. These efforts appear to have been effective. The number of AIDS cases dropped 13 percent from 1999–2000, and from 1995–2000 there was an overall decrease of 64 percent in reported AIDS cases and an 85 percent reduction in cases of mother-to-infant transmission of HIV.

Eastern Europe

The HIV epidemic did not reach Eastern Europe until the mid-1990s. In 1995, in all of Eastern Europe, only 31,000 of 450 million people were infected. By 1997, about 190,000 adults were infected with HIV, and by the end of 2000 an estimated 700,000 people were living with HIV/AIDS throughout Eastern Europe. Intravenous drug use has been the primary source for the spread of the virus.

Ukraine and the Russian Federation have been the hardest-hit countries in Eastern Europe. These countries showed the steepest increase in HIV infection from 1996 to 1999. According to estimates by UNAIDS/WHO, the former Soviet Union, as well as the rest of Central and Eastern Europe, saw a one-third increase in the total number of HIV infections during 1999. In the entire eastern European region during 1998 and 1999, 90 percent of AIDS cases reported during that period were from the Ukraine.

In 1994 only 44 people in Ukraine tested positive for HIV. In 1996 more than 12,000 tested positive, and, in 1997, 15,000 more new infections were identified. In 2000, an estimated 250,000 people were living with HIV/AIDS in Ukraine. In the Russian Federation, the story is much the same. In 1994, 158 people tested positive for HIV; most of those cases were attributed to MSM contact, while only two of the cases were reported among injecting drug users (IDUs). In 1997, nearly 4,400 people tested positive, three times as many as in 1996. In 1998, four out of five newly diagnosed cases were reported IDUs. During 2000, an estimated 50,000 new cases of HIV infection were reported, far more than the 29,000 cases registered in the twelve years between 1987 and 1999. The proportions of the epidemic may be significantly underestimated since, by its own admission, the Russian system manages to register only a small proportion of all cases.

ASIA

Asia—home to two-thirds of the world's population—could eventually overtake Africa as the continent most affected by HIV. The HIV/AIDS epidemic arrived in Asia much later than in the rest of the world. Until the mid-1990s, HIV/AIDS was uncommon, but because the average incubation period is approximately 10 years, more people are now beginning to die from the disease. WHO estimates that the number of infected Asians exceeded 5.8 million at the end of 2000. Although no Asian country has reached the prevalence levels seen in sub-Saharan Africa, by 1997, HIV was well established on the Asian continent. Most people infected with HIV are drug injectors and sex workers.

Most countries in Southeast Asia have been hard hit, with the exceptions of Indonesia, Laos, the Philippines, and Sri Lanka. In those four countries, fewer than one in one thousand adults were infected in 1999. Most of the

Southeast Asian countries have not developed sophisticated systems for monitoring the spread of HIV, so estimates are often made using less information than in other regions of the world. In populous countries, small differences in reported rates can mean a large difference in the actual numbers of infected persons.

Thailand

According to the UNAIDS, the incidence of new HIV infections decreased in Thailand in 1996 and 1997. This decrease was primarily due to ongoing prevention programs designed to increase condom use among heterosexuals, discourage men from visiting brothels, and discourage young women from entering prostitution by offering them more education and advising them about other employment prospects.

The spread of HIV in Thailand had been almost unprecedented. Thailand's commercial sex industry is notorious. In the capital city of Bangkok, brothels are found in virtually every neighborhood; and travel packages based on the availability of sex workers in Thailand are common in Asia. A 1990 survey found that 20 percent of all Thai men reported they had paid for sex in the previous year. After a military coup in 1991, the transitional government instituted a comprehensive AIDS education program, which included a media campaign and condom distribution to brothels and massage parlors. Brothels that refused to use condoms were closed down. While the anti-HIV program came too late for those infected in the mid- to late 1980s, Thailand recorded a drop in new HIV infections until the late 1990s.

Unfortunately HIV appears to be spreading among other high-risk groups, such as IDUs and MSM, who have not received as much attention in prevention campaigns. In 2001, an estimated 2 percent of adult males and 1 percent of adult females in Thailand were living with HIV/AIDS. The majority of the 675,000 adults living with HIV/AIDS are believed to be sex workers, their clients, and IDUs. Even if effective prevention measures continue, the epidemic will claim 50,000 Thais every year until 2006. The HIV infection rate is expected to persist in excess of 1.5 percent among adult males. In addition, more than 90 percent of AIDS deaths will occur in persons aged 20–44, the mainstay of the workforce.

Other Southeast Asian Countries

In other parts of Southeast Asia, current statistics on the epidemic show different patterns. As mentioned above, Indonesia, Laos, the Philippines, and Sri Lanka still record low rates of HIV infection. The reasons for the low rates are not clear. Moreover, there are no guarantees that prevalence will remain low; and some early indicators suggest changing patterns of incidence and prevalence.

Cambodia is the hardest-hit country in the region, with an estimated prevalence of 2.8 percent of people infected in 2000. In recent surveillance studies, 1 in 30 pregnant women, 1 in 16 soldiers and policemen, and 1 in 2 sex workers tested positive for HIV. Condom use has become much more common, with sales rising from zero to one million units per month in less than three years. However, commercial sex is still very popular. In a recent survey, three-fourths of respondents in the military and the police force and two-fifths of male students reported visiting a prostitute in the previous year.

In Myanmar (formerly Burma), HIV infection among sex workers rose from 4 percent in 1992 to over 20 percent in 1996, and nearly two-thirds of IDUs are infected. Tests of pregnant women in six urban areas showed that approximately 2 percent were infected with the virus. UNAIDS estimates prevalence at about 500,000 HIV/AIDS cases in 2000 and projects the addition of as many as 55,000 adult cases per year by 2005.

India

In July 1996, at the International AIDS Conference in Vancouver, British Columbia, a UN official reported that India had emerged as the country with the most people infected with HIV. This news came as a surprise to many of the conferees because HIV was not detected in India until 1986. In fact, by the end of 1993, only 5,000 AIDS cases had been reported to WHO from all of Asia. In 2000, according to the UNAIDS program, about 5 million of India's 950 million people were HIV-positive. Little is known, however, about how the infection flourished so quickly.

Although surveillance is irregular, recent testing indicates that the virus continues to spread. In Pondicherry, in the southeastern area of India, about 4 percent of pregnant women have tested positive. Five states—Maharashtra, Tamil Nadu, Karnataka, Andhra Pradesh, and Manipur—reported prevalence rates higher than 1 percent. AIDS deaths were estimated at 350,000 in 2000 and about 500,000 are anticipated in 2005.

In March 1996, industrialists in India launched a nationwide campaign to educate their workers about HIV and help prevent its spread. Most of India's HIV-infected population resides in the cities, especially Bombay, the country's financial capital, and along trade routes lined with brothels that serve truckers. Robert Friedman wrote in "India's Shame" (*The Nation*, Vol. 262, No. 14, April 8, 1996) that India has approximately 100,000 female prostitutes, most of them indentured slaves, and more than 50 percent are believed to be HIV-positive. With a population of one billion, half of whom are illiterate, the task of instituting effective HIV education and prevention programs is a daunting one for the government.

China

The first HIV case in China was identified in 1985, but the disease did not begin to spread until the early

1990s, when changes in the structure of the economy produced an increase in drug use and prostitution. At the end of 1996 the government of China estimated that as many as 250,000 people were living with HIV/AIDS, approximately 10 percent of them teenagers. By the beginning of 1998, that estimate had doubled. By 1999 half a million Chinese were estimated to be HIV-positive, and by the end of 2000, the estimate had risen to 600,000. By March 1998, however, only 9,970 HIV infections were confirmed, up from 8,277 confirmed cases in September 1997.

There appear to be two major epidemics growing in China. One is among IDUs in the southwestern portion of the country; the other, newer epidemic is among heterosexuals along the eastern seaboard. Prostitution along the eastern coast of China is growing as the gap between rich and poor widens. The number of reported cases of STDs has escalated sharply in recent years, a sure warning sign of the high-risk behavior that leads to HIV/AIDS. Paid blood donations are on the rise as well, and this is also fueling the rapid spread of the virus.

In 1997, the United Nations gave China a $1.8 million grant to help fight the disease over a four-year period. The funds were used to train ministry workers and to increase prevention education among high-risk populations. Although HIV education programs are common in urban areas, they have not reached the rural areas, where, when questioned, one-third of medical workers could not explain how HIV was transmitted.

Estimates of Chinese AIDS deaths in 2005 range from 60,000–100,000. Most of these will likely occur in the provinces where HIV prevalence is already high—Yunnan, Xinjiang, Guangxi, and Sichuan.

Overall about 6.5 million people are currently believed to be living with HIV in Asia and the Pacific—about 18 percent of the world's total cases. The huge populations of India and China dominate any assessment of HIV. Because the countries have so many inhabitants, small percentage changes in the estimates of national infection rates result in large changes in the estimates of the total number of people infected. For example, a rise of just 0.1 percent prevalence among adults in India would add over a half million people to the national total of adults living with HIV.

LATIN AMERICA

Initially, the majority of HIV/AIDS cases in Latin America could be traced to MSM transmission. More recently, the greatest increases have been among IDUs, although there have also been increases attributable to heterosexual transmission. Levels of transmission among men who have sex with men in urban areas of Brazil, Mexico, Argentina, and Honduras range from 20

to 35 percent. There are also indications of high HIV infection rates among commercial sex workers in some areas. Infection rates among IDUs, as a rule, have reached or exceeded 30 percent. In Brazil, HIV infection rates among IDUs have been reported as high as 40 percent in Rio de Janeiro, 54 percent in Sao Paulo, and 57 percent in Santos.

The picture in Latin America is mixed. In some countries, prevalence is rising rapidly, but in other parts of Latin America, infection is falling or remaining stable. Nearly every country in Latin America now reports HIV infections. More than half of Latin American countries report concentrated epidemics. These include the most heavily populated countries in the region: Brazil and Mexico.

The spread of HIV in Latin America follows the pattern of industrialized countries. Men who have sex with men and IDUs who share needles make up the highest risk groups. Studies done in Mexico indicate that about 14 percent of MSM may be living with HIV. Between 3 percent and 11 percent of IDUs in Mexico are infected; and in Argentina and Brazil, the proportion may be closer to half.

Rates are rising for women, indicating that heterosexual transmission is increasing. In 1986, one in seventeen AIDS cases in Brazil was a woman; in 1997 the number was one in four—one-fourth of the 550,000 adults living with HIV in Brazil were women. In Latin American during 2000, about 210,000 adults and children became HIV-infected and an estimated 1.8 million are believed to be living with HIV/AIDS. About one-fifth of those infected are women.

Several Latin American countries are beginning to establish programs to help care for those living with HIV/AIDS, including programs providing life-prolonging antiretroviral drugs. For example, in Brazil more than 85,000 people with HIV received government-subsidized antiretroviral therapy during 2000. Although overall access to care is better in Latin America than in most other areas of the developing world, it is not consistent throughout the region.

THE CARIBBEAN

In 1982, the first suspected AIDS cases in the Caribbean appeared in Jamaica. Since then, the epidemic has changed from a mostly homosexual phenomenon to a heterosexual one, with 65 percent of reported cases resulting from heterosexual transmission. About 35 percent of all HIV-infected adults in the Caribbean are women; and the prevalence rate among pregnant women has been rising each year. Unlike in other parts of the world, in the Caribbean the connection between HIV and IDU is low. But the rapidly growing popularity of crack cocaine and the traditionally common practice of men (and, more recently, women) having multiple sexual partners are fueling the spread of HIV.

Throughout the Caribbean, countries are confronting an epidemic that has left the region with the world's second highest incidence rate after sub-Saharan Africa. In 2000, according to UNAIDS, Haiti was the Caribbean nation hardest hit; about 8 percent of adults in urban areas and 4 percent in rural areas were infected, as were 13 percent of pregnant women who were anonymously tested. In the Bahamas, the prevalence rate among adults is 4 percent. In Trinidad and Tobago, 1 adult in 100 is infected, while in the Dominican Republic 1 in 40 is HIV-infected.

A number of factors contribute to these high prevalence rates:

- For many years, some Caribbean governments did not want to admit the problem for fear of losing their tourist trade.

- The area has seen years of political and social unrest.

- There are high poverty rates and low levels of education.

- Many Caribbean communities are vulnerable because of their socioeconomic disadvantages and lack of information.

- Migration between countries and from rural to urban areas contributes to the continued spread of HIV and makes it harder to prevent.

- There is little tolerance for MSM in the Caribbean, which means that many governments were unwilling to fight the disease until recently, when officials realized that most HIV/AIDS patients in the Caribbean were heterosexuals.

THE MIDDLE EAST

Less is known about HIV infection rates in North Africa and the Middle East than in other regions of the world. Middle Eastern countries with large numbers of immigrant workers carry out mass screenings for the virus, but no estimate places the number of infections at more than 1 adult in 100. The infection rate is estimated to be a low .13 percent; approximately 220,000 adults and children are thought to be living with HIV in these countries. Djibouti has reported that approximately 12 percent of its adults are infected—the highest adult prevalence in the region.

Because social and political attitudes in the Middle East and North Africa are generally conservative, it has proven difficult for governments to deal with risky behavior directly. Nonetheless, there are some community and non-governmental organizations that help sex workers and IDUs whose behaviors put them at risk for HIV infection.

WHO reports that in Middle Eastern countries, HIV/AIDS is viewed as a social stigma associated with MSM, a practice strongly disapproved of by the cultures and religions of the region. A large number of North African and Middle Eastern countries cannot be classified because of lack of data. Although limited data is available, there are indications that extensive spread of HIV has begun in some parts of North Africa and the Middle East, with 18 percent of adult deaths from infectious disease resulting from HIV/AIDS. The epidemic in the Middle East was just beginning in 1998, but there is some evidence that HIV infections are increasing among IDUs in Bahrain and Egypt. Although drug use is also frowned upon in these strictly religious, conservative cultures, trade in addictive drugs such as heroin appears to be substantial in some parts of the region.

CHAPTER 11

KNOWLEDGE, BEHAVIOR, AND OPINION

CONCERNS ABOUT HIV/AIDS

The American public appears less concerned about HIV/AIDS and its impact on health care than ever before. In 1988 more than two-thirds of all Americans named AIDS as the most urgent health problem facing the country. In 1993, 41 percent identified AIDS as the most pressing problem and another 30 percent named health care costs. In 1997, 29 percent of poll respondents cited AIDS as the most urgent health problem, 15 percent named cancer, and another 15 percent cited health care costs.

The 2000 Gallup poll marked the first time since 1987 that AIDS did not top the list of Americans' health care concerns; instead it came in third, trailing health care costs and cancer. In 2000 just 18 percent of Americans considered AIDS the most urgent health problem. Among young Americans aged 13–17, AIDS was rated the second most urgent health problem plaguing the country. Fourteen percent of young Americans cited AIDS, while 16 percent named cancer the number one problem. By October 2001 AIDS dropped even lower on the list of Americans' concerns as they focused on the more immediate issues of the economy and unemployment, terrorism, fear of war, and national security.

Over time people have grown less concerned about personally acquiring AIDS. In October 1997, according to *Gallup Poll Monthly*, 30 percent expressed some concern about getting the disease, down from 42 percent who felt that way in 1987. A Henry J. Kaiser Family Foundation survey conducted by Princeton Research Associates from August 14 to October 26, 2000 explored the attitudes, beliefs, knowledge, and opinions about HIV/AIDS. Using data provided by the Roper Center for Public Opinion Research at the University of Connecticut, the survey of 2683 adults found only 19 percent of respondents "very concerned" about becoming HIV-infected, and an additional 18 percent said they were "somewhat concerned." Thirty-nine percent of survey respondents reported that

they were "not at all concerned" about becoming infected with HIV.

Some attitudes about HIV have not changed a great deal. When asked if they were more or less concerned about a son or daughter becoming infected with HIV than they were a few years ago, 47 percent of respondents to the Kaiser Family Foundation Survey said they were "about as concerned." A similar proportion (50 percent) reported that they were "about as concerned" that they themselves would become infected as they were a few years ago. The remainder were about evenly divided between feeling more concerned (22 percent) and less concerned (25 percent) about becoming infected.

KNOWLEDGE AND TOLERANCE GROW

During the more than two decades since the virus that causes AIDS was first identified, aggressive community health education and awareness programs have sought to increase the public's knowledge about HIV/AIDS. Based on the findings of the 2000 Kaiser Family Foundation survey, American adults are better informed than ever before about HIV/AIDS.

The majority of persons surveyed (89 percent) know that presently there is no cure for AIDS and there are no drugs available that cure HIV (88 percent). Almost as many (79 percent) are aware that there is not yet a vaccine that protects against getting HIV.

In 1998 Americans were slightly more tolerant of those who contracted AIDS than they were in 1988. In 1987, 43 percent believed that AIDS was a punishment for the decline in moral standards. In 1997, 31 percent of those questioned felt that way. In 1997, 40 percent of poll respondents said that people have themselves to blame if they get AIDS, down from 51 percent in 1987.

Further evidence of increasing tolerance and decreasing stigma associated with HIV was the Kaiser Family

Foundation survey finding that about two-thirds of respondents believed they would not be thought badly of if people found out they had been tested for HIV. Fifty-two percent said they would be "not at all concerned" that people would think less of them if it was discovered they had been tested for HIV. An additional 13 percent said they would not be too concerned if people found out they had been tested for HIV.

Preventing HIV/AIDS

One of the biggest changes in the way Americans view HIV/AIDS today are the actions they take to prevent becoming infected with HIV. In 1997, only 15 percent of poll respondents said that they avoided associating with people who might have HIV/AIDS, down sharply from 43 percent in 1987. In 1997, 12 percent said they did not use public restrooms in order to lessen their chances of coming into contact with the virus, compared with 28 percent the previous decade. In 1997, 33 percent of Americans said they would avoid elective surgery requiring blood transfusions due to concern over the blood supply in hospitals, compared with the 42 percent who felt that way in 1987.

One of the most extreme measures of preventing exposure to HIV would be to isolate persons with HIV/AIDS from the rest of society. In 1997 only 7 percent of respondents supported that proposal, down significantly from 21 percent in 1987.

Along with taking precautions so they themselves do not acquire HIV, persons responding to the Kaiser Foundation survey expressed support for other measures to prevent the spread of HIV/AIDS. Fifty-eight percent favored needle exchange programs that offer clean needles to intravenous drug users (IDUs) in exchange for used needles, and 60 percent feel state and local governments should be permitted to use federal funds for needle exchange programs. A comparable proportion (61 percent) would allow IDUs to purchase clean needles from licensed pharmacists and 60 percent said physicians should be able to offer IDUs prescriptions for clean needles.

Preventing the spread of HIV is important to the persons surveyed. Nearly all feel that research to develop a vaccine to prevent HIV infection should be a priority of the federal government; 83 percent considered it very important and another 13 percent felt it a somewhat important government responsibility. The survey respondents were divided about the top priority for the federal government—44 percent favored vaccine research and 41 percent chose AIDS prevention and treatment.

TEEN ATTITUDES

Teens are worried about HIV/AIDS; the majority views it as a serious problem for their generation. In 2000, 34 percent said they were very concerned about becoming infected. This finding is from The Kaiser Family Foundation's *National Survey of Teens on HIV/AIDS 2000* which looks at attitudes and knowledge about HIV/AIDS in a representative sample of teens ages 12–17. The national survey also found that more African American and Latino teens felt very concerned about becoming HIV-infected than white teens. (See Figure 11.1.)

The overwhelming majority (more than 90 percent) of teens surveyed know that sharing needles and unprotected sexual intercourse place them at risk of HIV infection. This may reflect the fact that more schools, churches, synagogues, youth groups, and the media as well as parents are teaching students about HIV/AIDS and informing them about how the disease is spread. Still, not all teens are fully aware of the health behaviors that place them at risk; only 69 percent identified oral sex as a risk and just 41 percent knew that having another sexually transmitted disease (STD) increased the risk of HIV infection. (See Figure 11.2.)

Though they may be better informed because they have grown up with the HIV/AIDS epidemic, teens want to know more about HIV/AIDS and how it is spread, (48 percent) and where to get HIV testing (55 percent). More than half (57 percent) of the teens surveyed want to learn how to protect themselves from HIV infection and 46 percent want to know how to talk to a partner about HIV/AIDS. Slightly fewer teens (40 percent) want instruction about how to talk with their parents about HIV/AIDS and 36 percent would like to learn the proper way to use condoms. (See Figure 11.3).

African American and Latino teens and teen girls of all races and ethnicities reported the highest levels of interest in learning more about HIV/AIDS. Although many teens have been touched by the epidemic, and overall one in six teens said they knew someone who had tested positive for HIV, had AIDS, or died from AIDS, among African American and Latino teens one in four knew someone affected by HIV.

MISINFORMATION PERSISTS

Researchers have found that about half of American adults erroneously believe that drinking from the same glass as an HIV-positive person can transmit the virus, and about three-fourths of American adults think that immigrants and pregnant women, and others at risk, should be routinely tested for HIV infection. The research, conducted by Dr. Gregory Herek, a psychologist at the University of California at Davis, and supported by grants from the National Institute of Mental Health (NIMH), was described at the 12th World AIDS Conference in Geneva, Switzerland, in July 1998.

The research also indicated that along with incorrect ideas about how the disease is spread, instead of the declining stigma associated with AIDS reported by other

FIGURE 11.1

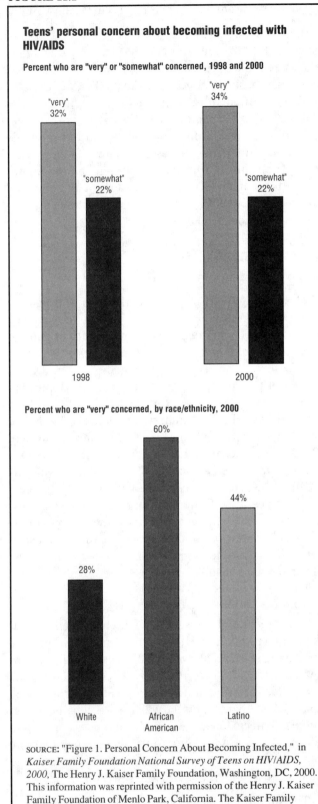

Teens' personal concern about becoming infected with HIV/AIDS

Percent who are "very" or "somewhat" concerned, 1998 and 2000

Percent who are "very" concerned, by race/ethnicity, 2000

SOURCE: "Figure 1. Personal Concern About Becoming Infected," in *Kaiser Family Foundation National Survey of Teens on HIV/AIDS, 2000,* The Henry J. Kaiser Family Foundation, Washington, DC, 2000. This information was reprinted with permission of the Henry J. Kaiser Family Foundation of Menlo Park, California. The Kaiser Family Foundation is an independent health care philanthropy and is not associated with Kaiser Permanente or Kaiser Industries.

FIGURE 11.2

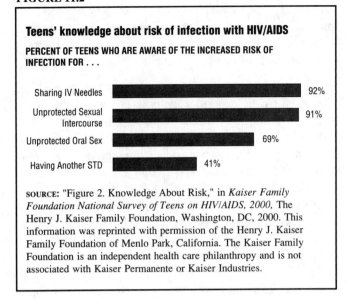

Teens' knowledge about risk of infection with HIV/AIDS

PERCENT OF TEENS WHO ARE AWARE OF THE INCREASED RISK OF INFECTION FOR . . .

SOURCE: "Figure 2. Knowledge About Risk," in *Kaiser Family Foundation National Survey of Teens on HIV/AIDS, 2000,* The Henry J. Kaiser Family Foundation, Washington, DC, 2000. This information was reprinted with permission of the Henry J. Kaiser Family Foundation of Menlo Park, California. The Kaiser Family Foundation is an independent health care philanthropy and is not associated with Kaiser Permanente or Kaiser Industries.

FIGURE 11.3

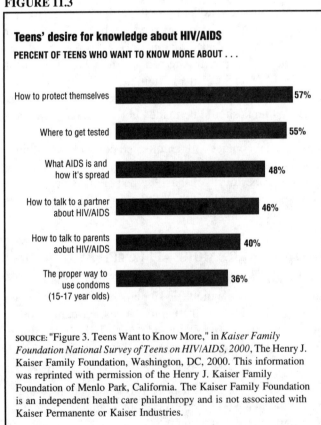

Teens' desire for knowledge about HIV/AIDS

PERCENT OF TEENS WHO WANT TO KNOW MORE ABOUT . . .

SOURCE: "Figure 3. Teens Want to Know More," in *Kaiser Family Foundation National Survey of Teens on HIV/AIDS, 2000,* The Henry J. Kaiser Family Foundation, Washington, DC, 2000. This information was reprinted with permission of the Henry J. Kaiser Family Foundation of Menlo Park, California. The Kaiser Family Foundation is an independent health care philanthropy and is not associated with Kaiser Permanente or Kaiser Industries.

surveys, the stigma surrounding the disease might be on the rise. According to Dr. Herek's random telephone poll of 1,712 adults in 1997, 29 percent thought that anyone who contracted AIDS through drug use or sex had "gotten what they deserve," up from 20 percent of people in 1991. The percentage of those who thought HIV could be spread by a shared drinking glass actually climbed from 48 percent in 1991 to 55 percent in 1997.

Fifteen years after the disease began to spread in the United States, it was still greatly misunderstood. More than one-fourth (27 percent) of those surveyed said they would be less likely to wear a sweater that had been worn once by a person with AIDS, even if the sweater had been cleaned and stored in a sealed package. One-third said they would not shop in a grocery store owned by someone who had AIDS.

Many of the conference attendees were surprised and disturbed by the results of the poll, especially the strong support for policies with the potential to increase discrimination against people believed at high risk of infection. One explanation offered for this persisting high level of misinformation is that most HIV/AIDS education is geared toward populations at high risk and not the general population. According to Wes Kennedy, education coordinator for the AIDS Prevention Project at the University of Texas Southwestern Medical Center at Dallas, Texas, people who do not see themselves at risk may not be as receptive to public health education. But he agreed that the fact that so many people continue to believe old myths is frightening.

HIV/AIDS experts and patient advocates were somewhat encouraged to learn that public support for the strictest anti-AIDS proposals seems to be diminishing. Dr. Herek's survey revealed that in 1997, 17 percent said they supported quarantining infected people, while in 1991, 36 percent felt that way. In addition, in 1997 only 19 percent of survey participants said they believed that the names of AIDS patients should be made public, compared with 30 percent in 1991. In 1997 fewer people said they would avoid social contact with an infected co-worker, and most agreed that AIDS patients are unfairly treated by society. However, one-fourth of the 1997 respondents agreed with the idea that people with AIDS are reckless and do not care about infecting others.

HISPANICS ARE MORE AFFECTED BY HIV/AIDS

Hispanics comprise about 13 percent of the population, but had accounted for 19 percent of all AIDS cases diagnosed by 2000 in the United States. Hispanic women are seven times more likely to become HIV-infected than non-Hispanic white women and almost one in four children under age 13 diagnosed with AIDS is Hispanic.

In May 1998 the Kaiser Family Foundation conducted a nationwide telephone survey in Spanish and English. One half of Hispanics surveyed believed AIDS was America's most serious health problem, and two-thirds said that HIV/AIDS was a serious problem for someone they knew. When compared with the overall adult population, nearly twice as many Hispanics said that they were "very worried" about becoming infected with HIV (24 and 46 percent, respectively).

According to the survey, most Hispanics (98 percent) knew that HIV/AIDS is a sexually transmitted disease, and 92 percent were aware that a pregnant woman could pass the infection on to her baby. However, only 77 percent knew that there is no cure for AIDS, and even fewer (68 percent) were aware that there is no vaccine against HIV.

Jane Delgado, president of the National Coalition of Hispanic Health and Human Service Organizations, emphasized that prevention strategies and education approaches must be tailored to address HIV/AIDS-related problems particular to individual communities. (For example, most Hispanics living in the northeast were infected with HIV through intravenous drug use, while men having sex with men was the major infection cause among Hispanics in Florida, California, and the Southwest.) Ms. Delgado also sees a need to adapt education and prevention materials so that people from all backgrounds can understand them.

PEOPLE WITH HIV/AIDS

Feeling Better

Despite regimens of potent antiretroviral drugs, 60 percent of HIV/AIDS patients surveyed reported that they are feeling good and rated their overall health as good or excellent. Speaking at the annual meeting of the Infectious Disease Society in San Francisco, Dr. Daniel Kaswan of the Infectious Disease Clinic at Montefiore Medical Center in New York presented the findings of a survey he and other researchers conducted in 2001. The researchers interviewed 80 men and 80 women who were HIV-infected and receiving treatment at the Infectious Disease Clinic. Even among the 60 percent of survey participants who had been diagnosed with AIDS, 70 percent said their health had improved over the past year. Two other findings also surprised the researchers—most patients (70 percent) could accurately predict the results of their laboratory tests and even those with full-blown AIDS rated their health as good.

HIV-Infected Males

Behaviors chiefly associated with increased risk for sexual transmission of HIV by infected people include unprotected sex and intravenous drug use. A CDC report in *Morbidity and Mortality Weekly* ("Continued Sexual Risk Behavior Among HIV-Seropositive Drug-Using Men," Vol. 45, No. 7, February 23, 1996) concluded that some HIV-infected men have relaxed attitudes concerning their HIV status. According to the report, they lack the motivation and knowledge to maintain safe behaviors that would decrease the risk of HIV transmission.

The survey, conducted in Atlanta, Georgia, Washington, D.C., and San Juan, Puerto Rico, found that some HIV-infected men continue to participate in high-risk behaviors. The 116 men interviewed were between the ages of 22 and 54 and reported being HIV-positive and sexually active. All the respondents also said they had used injected drugs or non-injected cocaine during the previous year.

Thirty-nine percent reported engaging in sexual activity with two or more partners, 28 percent reported vaginal or anal sex without a condom, and 23 percent said they had traded sex for drugs or money. A total of 37 (32 percent) had not informed their sex partners of their HIV status, and 73 (63 percent) did not know their partners' HIV status.

The 32 men who reported having unprotected sex were significantly more likely than those who used condoms to report multiple sex partners, having oral sex, trading sex for money or drugs, failing to disclose HIV status, and having intercourse more than 12 times during the previous month. These men were at a high risk of infecting their partners and reported an average of four sex partners with an average of 14 unprotected sex acts in the 30 days preceding the interview.

FAILING TO INFORM A PARTNER

Between 1994 and 1996, researchers at Boston City Hospital and Rhode Island Hospital questioned 203 HIV-infected patients receiving treatment, 129 of whom reported sexual activity in the previous six months. Four of every 10 HIV-infected people surveyed at two New England hospitals failed to tell their sex partners about their condition, and nearly two-thirds of those did not always use a condom.

Those questioned were mostly poor IDUs who did not have a high school education. Persons with only one sexual partner were three times more likely to have told their partner than those who reported multiple partners. Predictably, those with supportive partners were more likely to disclose their HIV infection. Whites and Hispanics were three times as likely to tell their partners as were blacks. Of those who were sexually active, 46 percent were black, 27 percent were white, and 23 percent were Hispanic. Of those questioned, 41 percent were infected through injection drug use, 39 percent through heterosexual contact, and 20 percent through MSM contact.

Dr. Michael Stein, director of HIV medical activities at Brown University Medical School in Providence, Rhode Island, noted that previous surveys of MSM produced similar findings, especially the greater likelihood that a person with one partner would admit HIV status than would a person with multiple partners. According to Stein, the problem is not one of knowledge, but of personal responsibility.

Failure to disclose HIV status or delaying telling a sex partner may be related to an HIV-infected person's social support system; those without close family, friends, and established sex partners may be less likely to reveal their HIV status. Researchers Lea Trujillo, Megan O'Brien and their colleagues at Tulane's School of Public Health and Tropical Medicine interviewed 269 people treated in New Orleans HIV clinics during the summer of 2000. Of the 269 men and women surveyed, 52 percent were African American and 80 percent reported becoming infected through heterosexual contact.

Nearly three-quarters of those with regular sex partners reported that they had disclosed their HIV infection to their partners, and 70 percent told their immediate families. In contrast, only one-quarter of persons with casual sex partners said they had disclosed their HIV infection to their partners. Further, those who did not tell their partners about their HIV infection were less likely to use condoms than those who had disclosed their HIV status to at least one casual sex partner.

Presenting the study at the October 2001 annual meeting of the American Public Health Association, Megan O'Brien warned that people who look and feel healthy while taking antiretroviral drugs may mistakenly assume that this effective treatment is a cure. O'Brien encouraged health professionals to teach patients about the importance of disclosure and how to tell their sex partners about their HIV infection. She cautioned uninfected people that they "cannot assume partners will volunteer their HIV status" and reminded them that they must assume responsibility for practicing safe sex.

IMPORTANT NAMES AND ADDRESSES

AIDS Action
1906 Sunderland Place, NW
Washington, DC 20036
(202) 530-8030
FAX (202) 530-8031
E-mail: aidsaction@aidsaction.org
URL: http://www.aidsaction.org

AIDS Clinical Trials Information Service
P.O. Box 6421
Rockville, MD 20849-6421
FAX (301) 519-6616
(800) 874-2572
E-mail: actis@actis.org
URL: http://www.actis.org

AIDS Project
American Civil Liberties Union (ACLU)
125 Broad Street, 18th Floor
New York, NY 10004-2400
(212) 549-2500
FAX (212) 549-2650
E-mail: aclu@aclu.org
URL: http://www.aclu.org/issues/aids/
hmaids.html

American Foundation for
AIDS Research (AmFar)
120 Wall Street, 13th Floor
New York, NY 10005-3902
(212) 806-1600
FAX (212) 806-1601
(800) 392-6327
URL: http://www.amfar.org

Body Health Resources Corporation
250 West 57th Street
New York, NY 10107
URL: http://www.thebody.com

Centers for Disease Control
and Prevention (CDC)
1600 Clifton Road
Atlanta, GA 30333
(404) 639-3534

(800) 311-3435
URL: http://www.cdc.gov

Centers for Disease Control
and Prevention (CDC)
National AIDS Hotline
(800) 342-AIDS (24 hours a day,
7 days a week)
Spanish Hotline (800) 344-7432
(8 a.m. to 2 a.m. Eastern Standard Time)
URL: http://www.ashastd.org/nah

Centers for Disease Control
and Prevention (CDC)
National Prevention Information Network
P.O. Box 6003
Rockville, MD 20849-6003
FAX (888) 282-7681
(800) 458-5231
E-mail: info@cdcnpin.org
URL: http://www.cdcnpin.org

Food and Drug Administration (FDA)
Center for Drug Evaluation and Research
1451 Rockville Pike, #6027
Rockville, MD 20852
(301) 594-6740
FAX (301) 594-6197
URL: http://www.fda.gov/cder

Henry J. Kaiser Family Foundation
2400 Sand Hill Road
Menlo Park, CA 94025
(650) 854-5270
FAX (650) 854-4800
URL: http://www.kaisernetwork.org

House Energy and Commerce Committee
Subcommittee on Health and
the Environment
2125 Rayburn House Office Bldg.
Washington, DC 20515
(202) 225-4952
FAX (202) 225-1919
URL: http://energycommerce.house.gov

Human Rights Campaign
919 18th Street, NW, Suite 800
Washington, DC 20006
(202) 628-4160
FAX (202) 347-5323
E-mail: hrc@hrc.org
URL: http://www.hrc.org

National AIDS Fund
1030 15th Street, NW, Suite 860
Washington, DC 20005
(202) 408-4848
FAX (202) 408-1818
(888) 234-AIDS
E-mail: info@aidsfund.org
URL: http://www.aidsfund.org/java.htm

National Association of People with AIDS
1413 K Street, NW, 7th Floor
Washington, DC 20005
(202) 898-0414
FAX (202) 898-0435
E-mail: napwa@napwa.org
URL: http://www.napwa.org

National Association of Public Hospitals
and Health Systems
1301 Pennsylvania Avenue, NW, Suite 950
Washington, DC 20004
(202) 585-0100
FAX (202) 585-0101
URL: http://www.naph.org

National Hemophilia Foundation
116 W. 32nd Street, 11th Floor
New York, NY 10001
(212) 328-3700
(800) 424-2634
FAX (212) 328-3777
E-mail: info@hemophilia.org
URL: http://www.hemophilia.org

National Institute of Allergy and
Infectious Diseases (NIAID)
31 Center Dr., MSC 2520

Bldg. 31, Room 7A50
Bethesda, MD 20892-2520
(301) 496-5717
FAX (301) 402-0120
URL: http://www.niaid.nih.gov

National Minority AIDS Council
1931 13th Street, NW
Washington, DC 20009-4432
(202) 483-6622
FAX (202) 483-1135
E-mail: info@nmac.org
URL: http://www.nmac.org

Center for Women Policy Studies
National Resource Center on Women
and AIDS Policy
1211 Connecticut Avenue, NW, Suite 312
Washington, DC 20036
(202) 872-1770
FAX (202) 296-8962
E-mail: cwps@centerwomenpolicy.org
URL: http://www.centerwomenpolicy.org

National Women's Health Network
514 10th Street, NW, Suite 400
Washington, DC 20004
(202) 347-1140
FAX (202) 347-1168
URL: http://www.womenshealthnetwork.org

The Orphan Project
121 Avenue of the Americas, 6th Floor
New York, NY 10013
(212) 925-5290
FAX (212) 925-5675
URL: http://www.aidsinfonyc.org/orphan

UNAIDS
20 Avenue Appia
CH-1211 Geneva 27
Switzerland
(+4122) 791-3666
FAX (+4122) 791-4187
E-mail: unaids@unaids.org
URL: http://www.unaids.org

RESOURCES

The Centers for Disease Control and Prevention (CDC) in Atlanta, Georgia, a division of the U.S. Public Health Service (PHS), in its *Morbidity and Mortality Weekly Report (MMWR)*, offers the most current accounting of the HIV/AIDS epidemic. Articles used in this publication from *MMWR* include "Revised Surveillance Case Definition for HIV Infection, 1999" (vol. 48, no. RR-13, 1999), and "Update: Syringe Exchange Programs—United States, 1998" (vol. 50, no. 19, 2001).

The *HIV/AIDS Surveillance Reports*, prepared by the CDC, are now published twice per year. In 2000, *Surveillance* included details of transmission categories, risk factor combinations, demographics, persons living with HIV, and the number of health care professionals who tested positive for HIV and AIDS through December 1997. Other CDC publications used to prepare this publication include *The 1993 Expanded AIDS Surveillance Case Definition* (1993) and *The 1994 Revised Classification System for Human Immunodeficiency Virus Infection in Children Less Than 13 Years of Age* (1994).

The National Center for Health Statistics (NCHS) in Hyattsville, Maryland, a division of the U.S. Public Health Service (PHS), publishes the findings from the *National Health Interview Survey in Advance Data*. Survey findings include "National Ambulatory Medical Care Survey: 1999 Summary" (Hyattsville, MD, 1999). The NCHS also provides an overall picture of the nation's health in its annual publication, *Health, United States, 2000* (Hyattsville, MD, 2000).

The Department of Justice, in its Bureau of Justice Statistics (BJS) *Bulletin, HIV in Prisons and Jails, 1999* (2000), includes information on HIV/AIDS in America's prisons and jails, inmate deaths from HIV/AIDS, and testing policies for the antibody for the virus by states.

Information on funding appropriated through the Ryan White CARE Act was published in *Ryan White CARE Act of 1990—Opportunities to Enhance Funding Equity* (Washington, D.C., 1995) and *HIV/AIDS—Use of Ryan White CARE Act and Other Assistance Grant Funds* (Washington, DC, 2001) by the General Accounting Office (GAO). The Health Resource and Services Administration Division of the U.S. Department of Health and Human Resources provided recent information on funding for the Ryan White CARE Act.

Information about the worldwide effects of HIV/AIDS, as well as projections for 2001 and beyond, were provided by reports from the World Health Organization and the United Nations Programme on HIV/AIDS (UNAIDS), both located in Geneva, Switzerland. The American Association for World Health (Washington, DC) also provides information and current facts on HIV/AIDS around the world and in the United States.

The Henry J. Kaiser Family Foundation publishes the results of surveys conducted by Princeton Research Associates using data provided by the Roper Center for Public Opinion Research at the University of Connecticut. The publication *Kaiser Family Foundation National Survey of Teens on HIV/AIDS, 2000* was used to prepare this publication. The Kaiser Family foundation also provides daily updates about a variety of issues related to HIV/AIDS at its online site http://www.kaisernetwork.org.

Information about many facets of HIV/AIDS may be found at the online site http://www.thebody.com. Several articles from the site were used in this report. The online sites http://www.biospace.com and http://www.home-drug-test.com provided information for this report on HIV home testing options. The status of pediatric AIDS was also covered in the report, using information in part from the Elizabeth Glaser Pediatric AIDS Foundation. The online Housing and Urban Development site (http://www.hud.gov) provided information on housing opportunities for people with HIV/AIDS.

Figures from *Confronting AIDS: Public Priorities in a Global Epidemic* (New York, 1997) by Oxford University Press and from *1998 World Development Indicators* (Washington, D.C., 1998) by the World Bank were helpful. In addition, figures and information from *AIDS Epidemic Update: December 2000* (Washington, D.C., 1999) were published by the World Health Organization and the United Nations Programme on HIV/AIDS (UNAIDS).

The Gallup Organization, Inc., publisher of the Gallup Polls, supplies timely data about public attitudes and opinions. We appreciate the Massachusetts Medical Society's tables from the *New England Journal of Medicine* article, "Physician-Assisted Suicide and Patients with Human Immunodeficiency Virus Disease" (Lee R. Slome et al., February 6, 1997). The Pharmaceutical Research and Manufacturers of America published the figure displaying pharmaceutical R&D spending in *PhRMA Annual Survey, 2001*.

INDEX

D

Dale and Betty Bumpers Vaccine Research Center (VRC), 76–77
Death benefits, 70
Deaths and death rates. *See* Mortality
Definition of AIDS, 1, 11–12, 12*t*, 13*t*, 15*t*–16*t*, 47–49, 48(*t*5.1)
Dementia, 14
Department of Defense testing, 87
Developing countries, 97(*f*10.2), 97(*f*10.3)
Diagnosis, 12, 48–49, 48(*t*5.2)
Discrimination, 80–81
Diseases
    leading causes of death, 2*t*, 3*t*
    opportunistic, 8–9, 11
Donation, blood. *See* Blood supply
Drug treatment. *See* Treatment
Drug use. *See* Intravenous drug use
Duesberg, Peter, 77

E

Early intervention services, 70
Eastern Europe, 102
Education, sexual health, 89–90
Elderly persons, 80
ELISA (enzyme-linked immunosorbent assay), 18
Emotional aspects, 80–83
Enzyme-linked immunosorbent assay (ELISA), 18
Europe, 101–102
Euthanasia, 83–84, 83*t*, 84*f*, 84*t*
Exposure categories
    AIDS cases by, 29*t*, 31*t*, 32*t*
    deaths by, 36*t*
    female adult/adolescent AIDS cases by, 32*t*
    female adult/adolescent HIV infection cases by, 38*t*
    heterosexual contact, 37
    HIV infection cases by, 50*t*
    HIV infection cases in adolescents and young adults by, 56*t*
    intravenous drug users, 37–40
    male adult/adolescent AIDS cases by, 31*t*
    male adult/adolescent HIV infection cases by, 39*t*
    pediatric HIV/AIDS cases by, 34*t*, 51*t*
    See also Transmission

F

Fauci, Anthony S., 6
Federal programs
    HIV-related care spending, 59, 67–70, 68*t*
    housing, 82
    syringe exchange programs, 93
Financial aspects of health care delivery, 59–63
Fisher, Mary, 79–80
Follicular dendritic cell network, 6
French blood supply, 17–18
"Friendly fire" theory, 5
Fusin, 6

G

Gallo, Robert, 3–4, 76
Gender
    adolescent and young adult HIV infection, 56*t*
    AIDS cases and rates by, 26*f*, 29*t*, 30*t*, 33(*t*3.10)
    AIDS deaths by, 23*t*, 36*t*
    HIV infection cases by, 50*t*, 54*t*
    office visits by, 61*t*
Gene research, 74
Generic drugs, 72
Genetic structure of HIV, 4
Geographic distribution
    HIV-positive inmates, 42
    international, 98–99
    metropolitan area case rates, 27*t*
    pediatric AIDS cases, 52–53, 52*f*
    regional differences, 24
German blood supply, 18
Grady Memorial Hospital, 63
Group for the Scientific Reappraisal of the HIV-AIDS Hypothesis, 77

H

Health care system
    assisted suicide, 83–84, 83*t*, 84*f*, 84*t*
    "Centers of Excellence" Program, 60–61
    financial aspects, 59–63
    health-care workers, 63–66
    home health care, 63
    Hospice care, 63
    hospital care, 61–63
    indigent patients, 61–62
    managed care networks, 60–61
    office visits, 61*t*, 62, 62*t*
    outpatient clinics, 63
    testing workers, 88
Health habits, 81
Hemophiliacs, 45–46, 57–58
Heterosexual transmission, 37, 98–100
Hispanic Americans
    AIDS cases and rates, 30*t*, 33(*t*3.9), 33(*t*3.10), 110
    AIDS deaths, 23*t*
    exposure categories, 31*t*, 32*t*
    female adult/adolescent HIV infection cases, 38*t*
    HIV infection cases, 54*t*
    male adult/adolescent HIV infection cases, 39*t*
    pediatric HIV/AIDS cases, 34*t*, 51*t*
HIV-2, 4
HIV (human immunodeficiency virus)
    antibody testing, 18–19, 47
    blood infiltration, 5–6
    development into AIDS, 7, 15–16, 19–20
    expanded surveillance case definition, 11–12, 12*t*, 13*t*, 15*t*–16*t*
    "Friendly fire" theory, 5
    fusin, 6
    identifying, 3
    link to AIDS dispute, 77
    molecular structure, 4
    mutation, 4–5
    origins, 3–4
    progression in children, 47

symptoms, 6
    the virus explained, 2–3
HIV-resistant gene, 74
Home Access Express HIV Test System, 19
Home health care, 63
Home testing, 19, 87
Homelessness, 57, 82
Hospice care, 63
Hospital care, 61–63
Housing, 82
HTLV viruses. *See* Retroviruses
Human immunodeficiency virus (HIV). *See* HIV (human immunodeficiency virus)

I

IL-12 (Interleukin-12), 7
Immune system
    cigarette and alcohol use, 7
    function of white blood cells, 4
    immunosuppression measurement, 11
    restoration, 7
    susceptibility to HIV, 6–7
    thymus gland, 75
India, 103
Indigent patients, 61–62
Infants, HIV-infected. *See* Perinatal infection
Insurance, 60, 70
Interleukin-12 (IL-12), 7
International data
    blood supply, 17–18
    effect of AIDS on birth and death rates, 97–98
    general discussion, 95–96
    life expectancy, 98*f*
    rates of infection, 1
    transmission means, 98–100
    trends and projections, 96–98
    tuberculosis, 99
    See also Individual countries
Intravenous drug use, 37–40, 45, 91–93

J

Johnson, Earvin "Magic," 79

K

Kaposi's sarcoma, 8*f*
    See also Cancer
Kenya, 100–101

L

Latin America, 104
Life expectancy, 98*f*
Life insurance, 60, 70
Long-term nonprogressors, 7
Louganis, Greg, 79
Lymph node infiltration, 6
Lymphadenopathy-associated virus (LAV). *See* Retroviruses

M

Macrophages, 4
Maine syringe exchange program law, 92
Managed care networks, 60–61
Mandatory testing, 85–86
Marrow cells, 6–7
Medicaid, 59, 70